# ARE Y...        ...RISK?

## THIS BOOK SEPARATES ...          ...FROM FICTION

## TRUE OR FALSE?

*"I see 20/20! I couldn't have glaucoma."*
False. Even people with perfect central vision can have (or develop) glaucoma. Most forms of glaucoma affect peripheral (side) vision first. Central vision is usually only affected late in the disease.

*"Ethnicity is a key risk factor."*
True. African Americans and Asians are at higher risk for developing glaucoma—and glaucoma is far more common among U.S. Hispanics than previously thought.

*"Glaucoma always leads to blindness."*
False. According to The Glaucoma Foundation, 90 percent of all glaucoma-related blindness may be preventable with proper treatment. That's why regular eye exams, early diagnosis, and treatment are so important.

*"People can get glaucoma at any age."*
True. Though its frequency increases with age, glaucoma can strike at any time in life.

*"I'd know if I had glaucoma because my vision would get worse."*
False. Most forms of glaucoma have no symptoms, and those affected often don't realize it until it is too late. Once vision has been lost to glaucoma, permanent damage has already been done to the optic nerve, and lost vision cannot be regained.

### NOW IS THE TIME TO LEARN . . .

# WHAT YOUR DOCTOR MAY *NOT* TELL YOU ABOUT™ GLAUCOMA

# WHAT YOUR DOCTOR MAY *NOT* TELL YOU ABOUT™
# GLAUCOMA

## The Essential Treatments and Advances That Could Save Your Sight

GREGORY K. HARMON, M.D.
with Nancy Intrator

Edited by Catherine Wang, M.D.

Foreword by Kitty Carlisle Hart

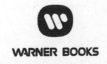

WARNER BOOKS

NEW YORK    BOSTON

This book is not intended as a substitute for medical advice of physicians. The reader should regularly consult a physician in all matters relating to his or her health, and particularly in respect of any symptoms that may require diagnosis or medical attention.

The title of the series *What Your Doctor May Not Tell You About* . . . and the related trade dress are trademarks owned by Warner Books and may not be used without permission.

Warner Books

Time Warner Book Group
1271 Avenue of the Americas, New York, NY 10020
Visit our Web site at www.twbookmark.com.

Printed in the United States of America

First Printing: October 2004

10  9  8  7  6  5  4  3  2  1

Library of Congress Cataloging-in-Publication Data

Harmon, Gregory.
    What your doctor may not tell you about glaucoma : the essential treatments and advances that could save your sight / Gregory Harmon with Nancy Intrator.
        p.  cm.
    Includes bibliographical references and index.
    ISBN 0-446-69062-7
    1. Glaucoma—Popular works. 2. Glaucoma—Treatment—Popular works. I. Intrator, Nancy. II. Title.
    RE871.H375 2004
    617.7'41—dc22                                              2004003580

*Book design by Charles A. Sutherland*
*Cover design by Diane Luger*

*This book is dedicated...*
*To my parents, John and Mildred Harmon, who have*
*encouraged and supported me every day, providing*
*me with a strong foundation upon which*
*to build my life and career*

*To my friend Kitty Carlisle Hart, who taught me by*
*example that personal success has real meaning*
*only through giving back to others*

# Acknowledgments

Many thanks to the very talented Rachel Ann Miller for creating many of the illustrations for this book.

I would also like to thank Dr. Catherine Wang and Jay R. Hoffman for their meticulous review of this manuscript and for their insightful comments, suggestions, and editing.

My special gratitude and most sincere thanks go to each member of my office staff for their help and support throughout the writing process and for their ongoing dedication to the patients who entrust us with their care:

Amalia Berdecia, medical secretary

Celenia Castaneda, medical clerk

Frank Fehr, ophthalmic assistant

Monique Flowers, medical clerk

Jenny Mai, O.D., clinical instructor of optometry

Kenneth Nieves, ophthalmic technician

Laritza Ramirez, C.P.C., account manager

Linda Reifschneider, medical secretary

June Maldonado-Resto, office manager

Melanie Sheinheit, O.D., clinical instructor of optometry

Christopher Spellman, M.D., Fellow in glaucoma and cataract

Minerva Suarez, ophthalmic technician, surgical coordinator

Margaret Trigueno, medical scribe

Zornita Vezenkova, M.D., pre-residency Fellow

# Contents

## PART III: RECENT ADVANCES

## PART IV: AN "EYE" TOWARD THE FUTURE

## PART V: WHAT YOU NEED TO KNOW NOW

# Foreword

If you are interested in your eyes, you should read this book.

About fourteen years ago, I was having my eyes examined, and the eye doctor thought my eye pressure seemed a little high. He brought me to see Dr. Harmon, who told me I had glaucoma. I didn't know it. I had no symptoms. I could have lost my sight. It could have been stolen away without the slightest indication it was on its way out.

Since then, Dr. Harmon and I have had many discussions about the importance of public education and eye health. In fact, we have done more than just talk. We created The Cornell Glaucoma Fund to raise money to increase the public's awareness of glaucoma and the importance of being tested for glaucoma. We filmed a public-service announcement that aired nationwide. I am told that people are still coming in to get tested because of that PSA. Dr. Harmon and I also appeared on television together to help spread the word.

But there is more outreach to be done. Half the people who have glaucoma still don't know it. That means they haven't had their eyes tested. Unless you have been tested, you can't know if you have glaucoma. If it turns out that you do have it, there are many ways you and your doctor can do something about it. This book will tell you all about those things. And if you

aren't convinced yet of the importance of getting your eyes
tested, you *will* be convinced after you read this book. Just
don't delay in making that call to your eye doctor to schedule
an appointment.

I'm ninety-three years old, and I have glaucoma. But I
haven't lost my sight. I haven't lost anything. That's because
once you know you have glaucoma, you can take steps to control it. That's what I did.

Pay attention to your eyes. You could lose your sight if you
don't.

*Kitty Carlisle Hart*

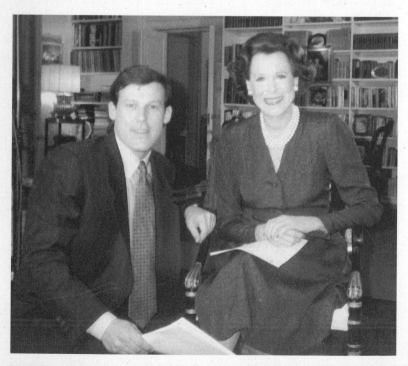

**Figure 1.** Kitty Carlisle Hart and Dr. Gregory Harmon in Manhattan during the filming of a Cornell Glaucoma Fund public service announcement
in May 1992. (Author's photo)

# Introduction

At first glance, the title of this book might seem to imply that I have some secret knowledge of glaucoma to share with readers. That their doctors might not be telling them everything they need to know about diagnosing and treating the "sneak thief of sight." That only *I* could tell them the truth without misleading them.

None of those implications are true. However, there are two factors that still make the title appropriate to the book.

First, the world of medicine, in general, is changing at a very fast pace. Many physicians no longer have the luxury of spending large amounts of time with patients, explaining all the ramifications of their conditions, explaining the reasoning behind treatment options, discussing alternatives, and responding to questions. Even if they do, patients today have learned to take a more active role in their own health care—as they should—and they often leave the doctor's office wanting more information, or they think of additional questions days after their appointment. It's not that your doctor doesn't *want* to tell you everything he or she knows about glaucoma, both during and after your appointment. There just isn't always the time for it. And at the time I agreed to write this book, there was no up-to-date consumer book on glaucoma on the market to fill the information void. This book is meant to supplement—not replace—the personal information your doctor provides.

Second, there is an explosion of new and exciting research in the field of glaucoma today. Although I am a glaucoma specialist myself, I still had to consult with colleagues, read an abundance of professional journals, and refer to textbooks in order to assemble all the information in this book. It took approximately two years to distill all this knowledge into a form that would be clear and understandable to nonphysician readers.* It would not be possible for any single physician to provide the same level of information to every patient who desires it.

It is the goal of this book to present exciting and vision-saving information that affects glaucoma management today. To communicate, as simply as I can, the information that my distinguished colleagues in glaucoma have assembled over recent years, through *their* research, clinical studies, and observations. To share the excitement I feel when I think about how much researchers and glaucoma doctors have really learned over the past few years. To get the message out that glaucoma is being better detected, treated, and understood than it was a few years ago. To tell the greatest number of people possible that they should get themselves screened for glaucoma on a regular basis and, if they are diagnosed with glaucoma, that they should follow their doctor's instructions to the letter. To help the nonphysician better understand why it is such an exciting time to be a glaucoma doctor. To give people a glimpse of what the future holds for people with glaucoma.

The future of glaucoma is a future filled with hope. Regardless of how much your doctor has told you, it's a message worth reading in full.

---

*For physicians: This book is written in the style common to consumer health books—*i.e.*, specific facts, figures, and studies are not footnoted and referenced within the text, but are referenced at the end of the book.

# Part I

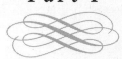

# UNDERSTANDING
# THE PROBLEM

# Chapter 1

# The Glaucoma Myths

How much do you know about glaucoma? What are the warning signs? Who is at risk? How is it diagnosed? Can you start losing your sight without knowing it? Is there any way to stop glaucoma? Can glaucoma damage be reversed?

Are your answers to these questions based on myth or fact?

The list of questions goes on and on. The price of not knowing the correct answers is high: Untreated, glaucoma can lead to blindness.

Most people can recite the warning signs of cancer. Just about everyone knows the risk factors for heart disease. But how many people know the facts about glaucoma?

Ask a fifty-year-old man about glaucoma and he might reply, "Only old people get glaucoma. I am young, and I have perfect vision. I don't need to worry about that." (Myth!) A person who believes that myth could go years without getting an eye exam. Now, imagine that this same man is age fifty, black, and diabetic. Since blacks tend to develop glaucoma earlier and more often, this man now has three serious risk factors for the disease—his age, race, and diabetes—and he doesn't even know it.

Here's another scenario: An elderly woman is diagnosed with glaucoma. She believes that glaucoma does not run in families. (Myth!) In this era of managed care, her doctor may simply not have enough time to sit down and explain that the disease is often hereditary and that other members of her family should be sure to have their eyes checked, regardless of their ages. Or maybe he will tell her, and she will just forget to pass along the message to her sons and daughters. Since her children are unlikely to know this fact about their own family history, they may be unknowing glaucoma victims for years, until a chance exam—or, worse, a deterioration in vision—reveals the diagnosis. (We will explore the relationship between eye pressure, glaucoma, and vision loss later in this chapter.)

Or maybe *you* have been diagnosed with glaucoma, and although you have followed your doctor's instructions regarding medication meticulously, the pressure in your eyes just isn't coming down or your vision is worsening. You wonder if there is anything more you can do without resorting to surgery. So you sign on to an online chat group for glaucoma patients. Someone tells you that jogging can reduce eye pressure. (Not a myth!) Another warns that wearing tight neckties can increase eye pressure and glaucoma risk. Really? (Not a myth!)

Since glaucoma is the leading cause of preventable blindness, we should *all* know the facts about this "sneak thief of sight." The first step is in knowing what *not* to believe. Learn how to separate myth from fact.

## THE MOST COMMON GLAUCOMA MYTHS

**Myth 1: All people with glaucoma have elevated intraocular pressure (IOP).**

Many people believe that glaucoma is a disease characterized and defined by elevated IOP. Actually, elevated IOP is a *risk factor* for glaucoma and is not the disease itself. The common thread among all glaucoma is *damage to the optic nerve* rather than elevated IOP.

There are more than forty different types of glaucoma, and not all of them are associated with elevated IOP. Glaucoma specialists believe that some forms of glaucoma are strongly related to vascular changes and impaired "nutrition" (poor blood flow) to the optic nerve.

**Myth 2: Only old people get glaucoma.**

Though its frequency increases with age, glaucoma can strike at any time in a person's life. In fact, glaucoma diagnosed in an adult may be a result of elevated intraocular pressure that began when that person was in his or her teens.

Approximately 1 in 10,000 babies is born with glaucoma, either because of a defect in the development of the drainage system of the eye or because of a congenital disease such as Marfan syndrome. Children between the ages of four and ten may develop a form of the disease called late congenital glaucoma, and for those affected between ten and thirty-five, the most common causes are hereditary disorders.

Individuals in certain high-risk categories may be more apt to become affected by glaucoma earlier in life. For instance, African Americans, who are six times as likely to suffer from glaucoma as Caucasian Americans, may begin to develop the disease in their forties (or younger).

## Myth 3: Glaucoma is always inherited.

Family history is a strong risk factor for glaucoma, but an absence of family history does not mean a person is risk-free. An individual's risk for glaucoma is increased by any and all of the following factors: elevated intraocular pressure; age over forty-five; Asian or African descent; diabetes; nearsightedness; high blood pressure; significant eye injury; and/or long-term use of cortisone or steroids. However, if there is a family history of glaucoma, everyone in the family—from children on up—should be sure to get regular eye exams.

## Myth 4: If you don't have high blood pressure, you cannot have high eye pressure.

Blood pressure and eye pressure vary independently. Controlling blood pressure does not mean IOP is controlled. However, high blood pressure is often—but not always—associated with elevated intraocular pressure. Interestingly, *low* blood pressure is strongly associated with some forms of glaucoma, such as normal-tension glaucoma (NTG).

## Myth 5: You can tell if you are developing glaucoma because your vision will deteriorate or blur.

Most forms of glaucoma have no symptoms or cause no change in vision until late in the course of the disease. Once vision has been lost due to glaucoma, permanent damage has already been done to the optic nerve, and sight cannot be regained. That is why early detection and treatment *before* vision loss occurs is so vital.

## Myth 6: You can test your own peripheral vision to see if you have glaucoma.

Most forms of glaucoma affect peripheral (to-the-side) vision rather than central (straight-ahead) vision. Many patients think that they can check their own peripheral vision by covering one eye, looking straight ahead with the other, and then checking to see what they notice at the side of their field of vision. On the basis of that type of "test," they decide that their peripheral vision is excellent and they could not possibly have glaucoma. However, it is impossible to evaluate the state of your vision without a true visual field test. That type of test is conducted in the eye doctor's office. Furthermore, as you will learn in the next few chapters, visual field testing is just one of the three vital diagnostic tests for glaucoma. It is also important for the doctor to look at the optic nerve head (disc) and to measure the IOP.

## Myth 7: Ethnicity has nothing to do with glaucoma risk.

Blacks and Asians are at particularly high risk for developing glaucoma. Researchers have also recently discovered that glaucoma is far more common among U.S. Hispanics than originally thought. Unfortunately, U.S. Hispanics have been found to be less aware of their increased glaucoma risk than are members of other ethnic populations, such as blacks.

Glaucoma also manifests itself differently in various ethnic groups. For instance, on average, blacks develop glaucoma ten years earlier than Caucasians. According to statistics from The Glaucoma Foundation, blacks who are between forty-five and sixty-five years of age and have glaucoma are fourteen to seventeen times more likely to go blind than their Caucasian counterparts. Furthermore, glaucoma is the leading cause of blindness among blacks.

**Myth 8: Nutrition and lifestyle have no effect on glaucoma.**

Other than taking their medication and going for eye checkups as directed, patients once believed that there wasn't much they could do to manage their own eye health. We now know this is not true. Nutrition, exercise, stress management, and other aspects of your lifestyle can affect every part of your body, and your eyes are no exception. Here are just a few of the latest findings:

• Research from the National Eye Institute (NEI) of the National Institutes of Health (NIH) has shown that the use of certain vitamin and mineral supplements can help preserve the health of certain structures within the eye. We have reason to believe that these substances may also help preserve the integrity of the optic nerve in glaucoma.
• Aerobic exercise such as jogging, swimming, brisk walking, or bicycling can help reduce IOP by as much as 20 percent if performed for at least thirty minutes, at least three times per week. Glaucoma patients should take care to avoid activities like scuba diving and yoga positions that involve standing on the head, since they can raise IOP.
• Smoking is associated with elevated IOP. Stop smoking.

**Myth 9: It is painful and time consuming to be tested for glaucoma.**

Nothing could be farther from the truth. There are three basic tests for glaucoma:

1. The **ophthalmoscopic exam**, in which the doctor looks into the eye and views the optic nerve.
2. **Tonometry**, in which a small instrument touches the front surface of the eye and measures the eye's pressure.

3. The **visual field test**, in which the eye is shown flashes of light that the patient is asked to detect in order to determine whether any side vision has been lost.

These tests are painless and relatively quick to administer.

## Myth 10: Your intraocular pressure is the same day and night.

Actually, IOP varies throughout the entire twenty-four-hour period, and these variations are more important than we previously thought. Patients with greater-than-normal variations in diurnal and nocturnal (daytime and nighttime) IOP are more likely to have progression of their glaucoma.

## Myth 11: Smoking marijuana is a good way to treat glaucoma.

For some people it might sound too good to be true: getting high under doctor's orders. It is true that clinical studies have shown that marijuana can lower intraocular pressure in individuals both with and without glaucoma. But does this mean smoking pot is an accepted and effective means of controlling glaucoma? The answer is a definite *no*.

The NEI initiated a number of clinical studies to determine the feasibility of marijuana as a form of glaucoma treatment. None of the studies showed the drug to be any more effective in lowering intraocular pressure than the Food and Drug Administration (FDA)–approved medications on the market. Furthermore, the active ingredient in marijuana has been shown to reduce blood flow to the eye. This reduced blood flow leads to a decrease in IOP. We now understand that adequate blood flow to the optic nerve is a critical factor in maintaining optic nerve health. Thus, the harmful effect of reducing blood flow to the eye negates the beneficial effect of lowering the IOP. In addition, studies showed that smoking marijuana could result in some potentially harmful effects such as increased heart rate and decreased blood pressure.

**Myth 12: If one medication does not lower my IOP, my doctor will add a second one and then a third until my IOP is controlled.**

Today there exists a large selection of safe and effective glaucoma medications. If the first one your doctor tries does not lower your IOP to the target level that has been chosen for you within a specified period of time, your doctor may *switch* you to a different medication rather than adding a second one to your regimen. It is much easier—and usually less expensive—for a patient to take one medication (monotherapy) rather than multiple medications, with a reduced chance of side effects. An easier treatment regimen enhances patient compliance. *In glaucoma treatment, compliance is key!*

**Myth 13: The target IOP should be the same for everyone.**

There is no one specific number that has been found to be *the* level at which a person's eye is safe from glaucoma-related damage. Some people require an IOP between 8 and 10 mm Hg while others can tolerate IOPs above 21 mm Hg. (Some basics: IOP is measured in millimeters of mercury. The abbreviation used is *mm Hg*. The normal range for IOP is considered 10–21 mm Hg.) Your doctor must be the one to choose *your unique IOP target level.* (The way your doctor chooses your IOP target level is discussed at length in chapter 6.)

## Myth 14: Glaucoma always leads to blindness.

This statement is one of the most dangerous of all the glaucoma myths. According to The Glaucoma Foundation, 90 percent of all glaucoma-related blindness could have been prevented with proper treatment. In fact, glaucoma is the leading cause of *preventable* blindness. But you can't get treatment unless you know you have a problem, and currently only about half of all the people who have glaucoma are aware of it. If everyone had regular eye screenings and all glaucoma patients were diagnosed in a timely fashion, got the appropriate treatment advice, and followed all the doctor's instructions regarding medication, lifestyle changes, and—if necessary—surgery, there is a good chance that the sneak thief of sight could be stopped and blindness avoided.

## Myth 15: If I have a cataract and glaucoma, I will need two separate surgeries.

There are times when patients who need both cataract and glaucoma surgery will require two separate surgeries, but this is not always the case. If a glaucoma patient is in need of cataract surgery, the doctor has three options: cataract surgery alone; staged surgeries (surgeries for the two conditions performed at different times); and combined cataract–glaucoma surgery. In chapter 9, I will describe these procedures and which patients are good candidates for each approach.

## Myth 16: When it comes to glaucoma treatment, there is nothing new to offer.

There is never a good time to be a glaucoma patient, but for individuals who do develop glaucoma, there has never been a time to be more optimistic. There is hope . . . and lots of it! We now have an entirely new class of drugs that makes treating glaucoma safer, easier, and more effective than ever before: the hypotensive lipids. New surgical techniques have been developed for improving drainage and lowering pressure within the eye. It is only recently that we have learned of the role nutrition and exercise can play in controlling IOP. Furthermore, only recently have researchers identified a new, potentially crucial risk factor for glaucoma: thin central corneal thickness (CCT). The discovery of this risk factor is already helping doctors identify patients at high risk for developing glaucoma. It is also helping doctors better understand and treat glaucoma in certain existing patients.

The future holds even more promise. Researchers have already identified a genetic marker for glaucoma. This could revolutionize screening and treatment techniques, possibly even preventing the onset of glaucoma in at-risk individuals. New methods of protecting the optic nerve (and thus preserving sight) in glaucoma patients are being developed. Researchers are experimenting with ways of suppressing an enzyme that produces retinal damage in glaucoma. Scientists are investigating the possibility of using stem cell technology to replace retinal cells that have been destroyed by glaucoma-related damage. Retinal implants that transmit digital images to the brain via a camera (attached to eyeglasses) allow previously blind patients to see movement and detect light and dark. Scientists are working on more advanced implantable devices that will provide greater vision to patients who have lost sight.

**Myth 17: I have great vision. I see 20/20! I don't even wear glasses. I couldn't have glaucoma.**

Even people with perfect central vision can have (or develop) glaucoma. Glaucoma usually affects peripheral vision first, rather than central vision. Central vision (visual acuity) is usually only affected late in the disease.

It is true that nearsighted people are at greater risk for developing glaucoma. It is also true that farsighted people are more likely to develop narrow angles and ultimately, primary angle-closure glaucoma. (You will learn more about the different types of glaucoma in chapter 4.) Overall, however, even if you have good visual acuity with or without glasses, you could still develop glaucoma!

The best way to gain control over glaucoma is to learn all you can about the disease so that you can debunk the myths. This book will give you all the information you need to do that.

Your first step will be to develop a good understanding of how the eye works, what goes wrong when glaucoma strikes, which individuals are most likely to be at risk, and the various forms glaucoma can take. This will all be covered in part 1: Understanding the Problem.

In part 2: Established Methods of Controlling Glaucoma, you will learn about the current, most up-to-date ways in which glaucoma is diagnosed and treated, including medications, laser surgery, and traditional surgery. You will also learn about current theories on the effects of nutrition, herbal therapy, exercise, stress reduction, and lifestyle on glaucoma.

In part 3: Recent Advances, you will learn about some true breakthroughs in diagnosis and treatment that have already been established and are in use across the country. Part 4 (An "Eye" Toward the Future) will describe promising, cutting-edge innovations currently in the research stage. Part 5 (What You Need to Know Now) will provide you with an overview of important steps you can take now to protect your sight.

After you have finished reading this book, you will be well informed and able to separate myth from fact regarding glaucoma, the sneak thief of sight.

*Chapter 2*

# The Healthy Eye

In order to understand the various forms of glaucoma, it is necessary to know how the eye works and become familiar with its structures. Many parts of the eye are analogous to those of a simple box camera. In fact, the way we see is not so very different from the way we take a picture (figures 2a and 2b). When you want to take a picture, the light that illuminates the subject passes through the aperture of the camera and becomes focused on the film behind the lens. Similarly, when you look at an object, the light illuminating it passes through the clear cornea at the front of your eye and through your pupil (the aperture of your "camera") and crystalline lens. The image becomes focused on the retina (the "film" of your camera), the transparent, interior surface of your eye that contains millions of nerve endings. It is from there that the picture of what you are seeing is relayed to your brain for processing via the 1.2 million axons of the optic nerve.

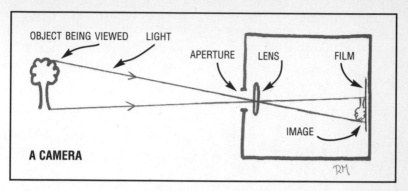

**Figure 2a.** How a camera takes a picture: Light illuminating the object being viewed passes through the camera's aperture, becomes focused by the lens, and is processed into an image on the film.

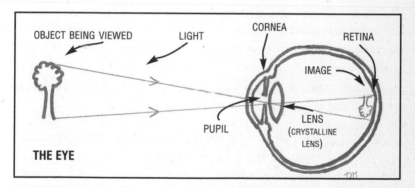

**Figure 2b.** How the eye sees: Light illuminating the object being viewed passes through the cornea and pupil, becomes focused by the crystalline lens, and is processed into an image on the retina.

The eye has three layers:

1. The outer fibrous layer, which consists of the cornea and the sclera.
2. The inner, or vascular layer, called the uveal tract. This consists of the choroid, the ciliary body, and the iris.

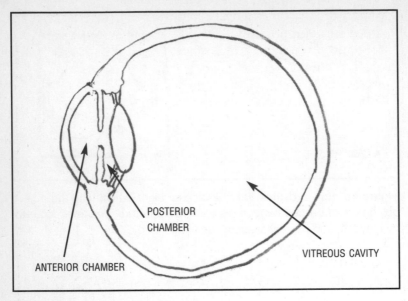

**Figure 3.** The chambers of the human eye.

3. The neurosensory layer, which is the innermost layer. This layer contains the retina.

We can also divide the eye (figure 3) into three chambers: the anterior chamber (in front of the iris), the posterior chamber (between the iris and the lens), and the vitreous cavity (behind the lens).

## THE PARTS OF THE EYE

The following are descriptions of the key structures of the human eye as depicted in figure 4 and discussed throughout this book. Please refer to figure 4 as you read this section.

• **Conjunctiva:** A semitransparent tissue that contains many blood vessels and covers the surface of the eyeball.

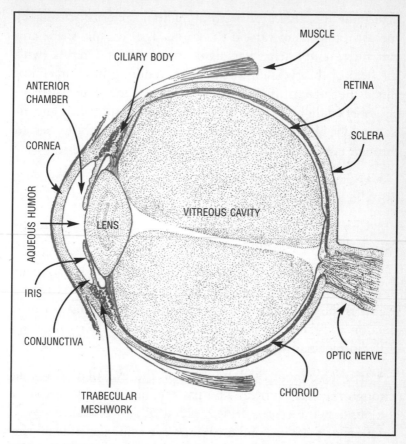

**Figure 4.** The anatomy of the human eye. (Courtesy of National Eye Institute, National Institutes of Health)

• **Sclera:** The thick, outer shell of the eye. It is whitish and opaque—what is commonly called the whites of your eyes.

• **Cornea:** The clear, outer portion of the eye through which light enters. The cornea helps focus light that enters the eye. Its specific shape and curvature, as well as the tear film, are the outermost focusing aspects of the eye. The curve and shape of the cornea are fixed, and it is these aspects of the cornea that determine the degree of focusing. The degree of focusing by the cornea does not vary. If the cornea is of normal shape and curvature, it will help focus light precisely on the retina (with the help of the eye's lens, of course), resulting in clear vision. But if the curve of the cornea is too steep, too flat, or irregularly shaped, light will not be well focused on the retina and vision will be blurry. This lack of focus (or blur) can be corrected through eyeglasses, contact lenses, or refractive surgeries.

• **Uvea:** A highly vascular area that consists of the choroid, the ciliary body, and the iris.

• **Choroid:** The vascular, middle coat of the eye, positioned between the sclera and the retina.

• **Ciliary body:** The structure that produces the aqueous fluid, which fills the anterior and posterior chambers of the eye. It is the dynamics of the aqueous humor (its rate of production and rate of drainage from the eye) that determine the IOP (intraocular pressure).

• **Iris:** The pigmented portion of the eye that is visible through the clear cornea. The iris acts like an aperture, with the pupil at the center. Irides (plural of *iris*) contain varying amounts of pigment, and a person's eye color depends on the specific amount of pigment in the iris. Brown eyes have the most pigment; blue eyes have the least.

• **Pupil:** The central aperture of the iris. The pupil varies in diameter depending on the amount of light present. In darker environments, the pupil dilates to allow more light to enter the eye. In bright light, the pupil becomes much smaller (constricted) reducing the amount of light that can enter the eye.

• **Aqueous humor:** The watery substance produced by the ciliary body. It provides the cornea and lens with nutrients and oxygen and helps maintain the necessary pressure for the eye to retain its shape. The aqueous humor can also be referred to as simply the aqueous.

- **Trabecular meshwork:** The part of the eye that functions like a drain: a small (one-fiftieth of an inch) piece of spongy tissue through which the aqueous humor drains into Schlemm's canal, ultimately leading into the veins of the eye and body. The trabecular meshwork is located where the iris and cornea meet (the limbus).

- **Schlemm's canal:** A channel contiguous with the trabecular meshwork. This is the conventional route of outflow for the aqueous humor.

- **Lens:** The crystalline lens lies immediately behind the iris. It is held in position by thousands of tiny fibers: the zonules. The lens focuses light for the eye. The lens is malleable, which means that it is capable of changing its shape. In a complex mechanism involving the muscles inside the eye and the zonules, the lens can become thinner or thicker, varying the amount of focusing that it does. It is the ability of the lens to change shape that allows us to accommodate—focusing on things that are near, as when you read this book. This ability to accommodate by way of the lens changing shape gradually reduces as we age. That is why we begin to need reading glasses in our midforties, even if distance vision is still perfect. (This is called presbyopia.)

- **Vitreous humor:** The gel-like substance that fills the vitreous cavity (area behind the lens). Like the aqueous, the vitreous humor can be referred to as simply the vitreous.

- **Retina:** The transparent, inner layer of the eye that contains the nerve cells that capture and transmit images to the optic nerve.

• **Optic Nerve:** A cranial nerve that contains 1.2–1.5 million axons (nerve fibers) and connects the eye to the brain. The optic nerve head is often referred to as the disc.

Since intraocular pressure (IOP) is a major risk factor for glaucoma and is often elevated in glaucoma patients, let's take a closer look at how aqueous fluid escapes from the eye.

Aqueous humor is constantly being produced by the ciliary body to nourish and oxygenate the cornea and lens. Naturally, there is an exit route for this fluid, creating a balance between fluid made and fluid exiting the eye. Otherwise, pressure within the eye would build to an unhealthy level. In a normal eye 90 percent of aqueous outflow is the *conventional* type and 10 percent of aqueous outflow is of the *nonconventional* type.

## AQUEOUS OUTFLOW: CONVENTIONAL

Conventional outflow of the aqueous humor is through the trabecular meshwork to Schlemm's canal, and on to the venous system of the eye (figure 5). The trabecular meshwork acts very much like a sieve; it is the amount of resistance that the aqueous encounters in its outflow path that determines the IOP. In other words, if the aqueous can flow easily through the eye's drainage system, IOP will probably be normal. If resistance to outflow is very high, however, the aqueous has a hard time exiting the eye, and IOP rises. If the trabecular meshwork is blocked, outflow will be affected, and IOP rises even more.

## AQUEOUS OUTFLOW: NONCONVENTIONAL

The other, nonconventional route of aqueous outflow is the uveoscleral outflow path (figure 6). This accounts for only about 10 percent of outflow in a normal eye.

In the nonconventional route, the aqueous—having been

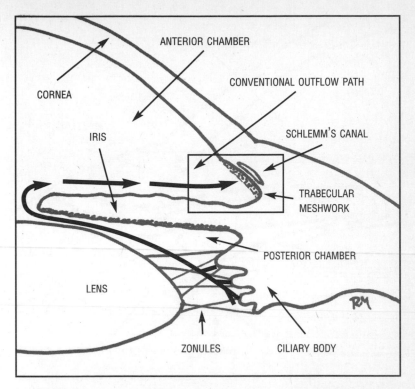

**Figure 5.** The conventional outflow pathway: Aqueous flows from the ciliary body through the posterior chamber, passing between the front surface of the lens and the posterior surface of the iris, entering the anterior chamber. From there, the aqueous exits the eye through the trabecular meshwork, enters Schlemm's canal, and goes into collector channels and the episcleral veins, thus reentering the venous circulation of the body.

formed in the ciliary body—passes from the anterior chamber into microscopic spaces within the ciliary muscle. It passes into the supraciliary-suprachoroidal space and then through the sclera or through the perivascular spaces of the emissary channels (small perforations in the sclera that allow nerves and blood cells to go through the sclera). The rate of flow depends

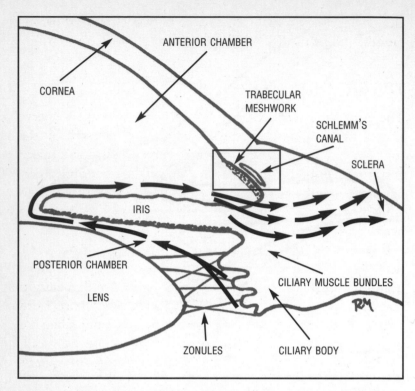

**Figure 6.** The nonconventional outflow pathway (uveoscleral outflow): Aqueous exits the eye by passing from the anterior chamber into microscopic spaces within the ciliary muscle and then through the sclera.

on the permeability of the ciliary muscle. Typically, aqueous flows at approximately 0.2 microliter per minute (which is 10 percent of total flow).

Uveoscleral outflow is largely pressure-independent at high IOP levels. In other words, when the IOP is greatly elevated, there is no significant increase in uveoscleral outflow. However, uveoscleral outflow appears to be pressure-dependent at low IOP levels. In situations where there is inflammation inside the anterior chamber of the eye (iritis), the spaces within the muscles of the ciliary muscle are enlarged, uveoscleral outflow increases, and IOP falls.

## THE OPTIC NERVE

The optic nerve is made up of 1.2 to 1.5 million axons (nerve fibers). It transmits the signals and impulses received by the retina to your brain. The optic nerve can be considered analogous to a massive cable that transmits signals to your television or connects to your high-speed Internet. Without that link to your brain, you would not be able to see—no matter how healthy the rest of your eye might be.

When the eye doctor looks into the eye, the entire optic nerve cannot be seen. Only the very top of it—the optic nerve head—is visible. The optic nerve head is only 1.5 millimeters in diameter. Each individual fiber (axon) carries information from a specific area of the retina. So, in glaucoma, as certain fibers are damaged, specific and related defects in the visual field are seen. Damage within a specific point of your visual field corresponds directly to damage within specific fibers of the optic nerve and its components. Remember this key point: Regardless of the type of glaucoma, it is damage to the optic nerve fibers that is the shared characteristic of all glaucoma, not elevated IOP.

As damage to the fibers of the optic nerve progresses, cupping of the nerve can be seen during the eye exam.

### What Is Cupping of the Optic Nerve?

As damage to the fibers of the optic nerve progresses, cupping of the nerve can be seen during the eye exam. To explain the concept of cupping of the optic nerve to my patients, I usually ask them to close their eyes and imagine a white teacup without a handle sitting on a bright red saucer. I then ask the patients to imagine placing that teacup and saucer down by

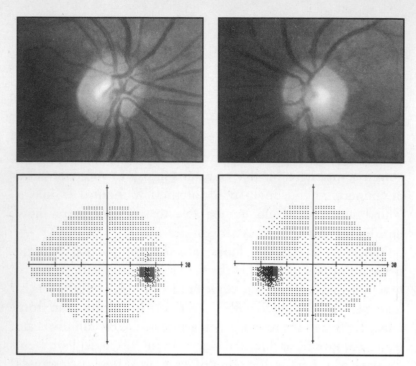

**Figure 7.** A normal optic disc and visual field (top row: right eye optic disc, left eye optic disc; bottom row: right eye visual field, left eye visual field): Note that the cup-to-disc ratio is approximately 0.3. A normal visual field has a blind spot located approximately 15 degrees from the center of the field of vision (fixation).

their feet. I tell them to look directly down onto that red saucer and white teacup. What they see is a red disc with a white center. The central part—the cup—has depth. The saucer surrounding the cup is evenly distributed all the way around the cup. The cup is probably about one-third of the total diameter of the saucer. This is what the typical optic nerve head looks like when the doctor looks into the eye. When looking at your optic nerve head, the doctor sees a red saucer with a pale, whitish central zone. This pale central zone is called the *cup*,

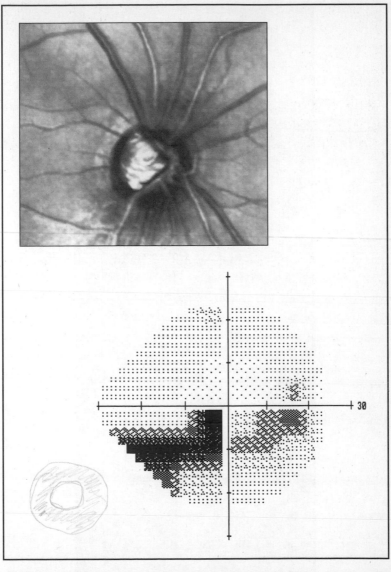

**Figure 8.** A glaucomatous optic disc and visual field (top: right eye optic disc; bottom: right eye visual field): Erosion (damage) of the superior (upper) part of the disc corresponds to a defect in the inferior (lower) part of the visual field.

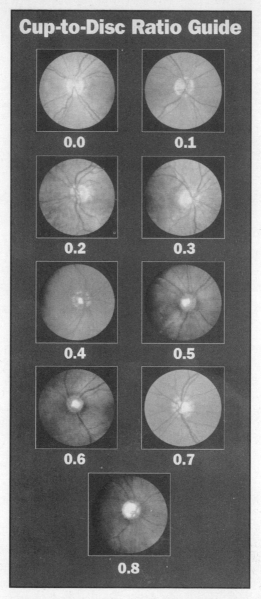

**Figure 9.** Cup-to-disc ratio guide: A higher cup-to-disc ratio may indicate glaucoma damage.
(Courtesy of Mansour Armaly, M.D.)

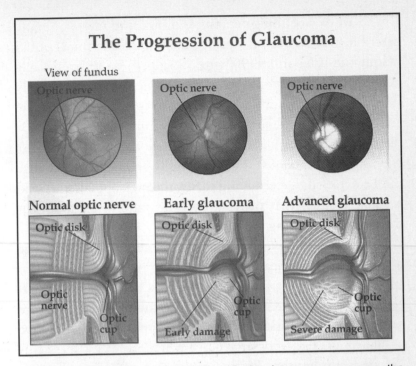

## The Progression of Glaucoma

View of fundus

Optic nerve

Optic nerve

Optic nerve

Normal optic nerve

Early glaucoma

Advanced glaucoma

Optic disk

Optic disk

Optic disk

Optic nerve

Optic cup

Optic cup

Early damage

Optic cup

Severe damage

**Figure 10.** The progression of glaucoma: As glaucoma progresses, the optic nerve head shows increasing cupping (excavation). In early stages, a small amount of cupping is seen; in advanced glaucoma, there is severe damage and associated severe cupping. The optic nerve head shows a cup-to-disc ratio of greater than 0.9. The blood vessels of the nerve head are displaced to the nasal side. Overall, the disc appears pale and excavated. (Copyright 1996 Humanatomy® Illustration, a registered trademark of Tim Peters and Company, Inc., Peapack, NJ 07977. All rights reserved. www.humanatomy.com.)

and the reddish saucer is referred to as the *disc*. The doctor judges what the cup-to-disc ratio is—how big the teacup is relative to the saucer. In the normal optic nerve head, the cup-to-disc ratio is about one-third. When the cup-to-disc ratio is greater than that, or is felt to be greater than normal, this is called cupping (see figures 7–10).

The art of describing cupping is difficult to master. Simply describing the cup-to-disc ratio as 0.3 (about one-third) or 0.5 (about one-half) or 0.9 (90 percent cupped) is only minimally helpful (but still useful). What is *more* helpful is to carefully sketch the nerve head, photograph it stereoscopically, or create an image of it using modern imaging techniques. These will be discussed in chapters 5 and 13. The more accurately a person's cupping is documented, the more easily any degree of change can be detected. Determining that someone's optic nerve head is stable requires that there be documentation over time that the degree of cupping and the visual field remain unchanged.

Despite the best possible information about the appearance of the optic nerve head and its cupping, the optic nerve can still appear to be cupped (and appear to be affected by glaucoma) when it isn't. This is especially true in people who are nearsighted. The optic nerve head can appear to be suggestive of glaucoma (with very large cups) when, in reality, it is actually perfectly healthy. *Remember this important fact: The appearance of the optic nerve head alone is insufficient in determining whether a person has glaucoma.*

## The Angle

Another important anatomical consideration involves the depth of the anterior chamber (front of the eye) bounded by the iris and cornea. The depth of the anterior chamber is usually directly related to the specific way in which the iris meets the cornea: the angle.

In a normal, healthy eye, the angle between the iris and cornea is approximately forty degrees. If the angle is smaller than normal, there is a higher risk of angle-closure glaucoma. I will discuss this in greater detail in chapter 4.

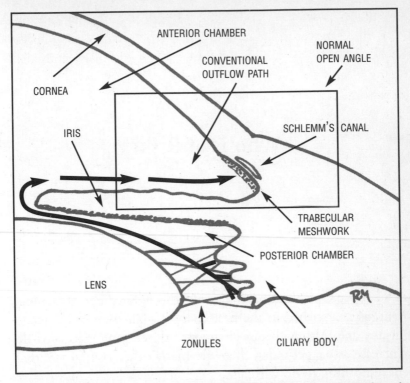

**Figure 11.** The normal angle: The angle is formed by the intersection of the iris and the cornea. The trabecular meshwork lies at that intersection.

*Chapter 3*

# Who Is at Risk?

Many people assume that only the elderly get glaucoma. But, as I described in the first chapter, glaucoma can develop at any age. Although our chances of developing glaucoma do increase as we get older, there are many other risk factors that have nothing to do with age.

It is very important to know whether you are in an increased-risk category or not. Everyone should be screened for glaucoma on a regular basis, but this monitoring is especially important for individuals who have one or more risk factors for developing the disease. In fact, as of January 1, 2002, Medicare covers the cost of glaucoma screening for individuals at high risk of developing glaucoma. High-risk Medicare beneficiaries include those who fall into any of the following categories: individuals with diabetes mellitus; individuals with family history of glaucoma; and individuals of African American descent.

Let's take a closer look at some of the known risk factors.

## ELEVATED INTRAOCULAR PRESSURE (IOP)

In the past, doctors believed that elevated IOP was synonymous with glaucoma. We now understand that a person can develop glaucoma without having elevated IOP, or can be free of glaucoma even though the IOP is elevated. Elevated IOP is a very significant risk factor for glaucoma, but it is just that: a risk factor. *It is not the disease itself.*

## AGE OVER FORTY-FIVE

Glaucoma can develop at any age. However, the risk does increase as you get older. Statistically, the point of increased risk begins at age forty-five. It is at this point that increased vigilance in terms of monitoring becomes especially important.

## FAMILY HISTORY OF GLAUCOMA

The important thing to remember when I refer to family history is that I mean *all* blood relatives. Patients tend to think only in terms of parents and siblings. Often a patient will say something like, "No, I have no family history of glaucoma. Just my maternal aunt and a cousin have glaucoma." Moreover, many people don't even know their family medical histories. I urge you to find out—not just about glaucoma, but about other medical conditions as well.

Once I diagnose a patient as having glaucoma, I encourage him or her to send in any and all family members—brothers, sisters, aunts, uncles, parents, and children—to be tested, and to spread the word throughout all branches of the family tree: *Get tested for glaucoma!*

## ETHNIC BACKGROUND

Ethnic background has a significant impact on both the degree of risk for glaucoma and the type of glaucoma that is most likely to develop. Being black increases the risk of developing glaucoma four- to sixfold. It is estimated that 1 in 13 blacks have glaucoma. Glaucoma in blacks also tends to be more aggressive than in people of other ethnic backgrounds. These differences are probably genetic in nature, but doctors do not know why blacks are at a much greater risk for glaucoma and glaucoma-related blindness than Caucasians. Studies indicate that black patients are likely to fare better with earlier, more aggressive treatment—earlier laser treatment, earlier surgery, and so on. Even with equivalent treatment and monitoring, however, blacks are more likely than Caucasians to lose their sight from glaucoma, since their glaucoma tends to be more aggressive. Glaucoma is also more common in Hispanics.

Asians are at higher risk for developing angle-closure glaucoma (ACG) and normal-tension glaucoma (NTG).

## DIABETES MELLITUS

Diabetes affects the eye in many ways, especially the retina and its blood supply. Any condition that potentially affects the blood supply to the nerve cells in the eye increases the risk of vision loss—including, but not limited to, glaucoma.

## NEARSIGHTEDNESS

Individuals who are nearsighted have a higher-than-normal risk of developing glaucoma. Most glaucoma doctors consider nearsightedness (especially significant or high degrees of nearsightedness) to be a risk factor for glaucoma because many (although not all) studies have found this to be true. A recent follow-up to the Beaver Dam Eye Study (a study designed to evaluate the prevalence of glaucoma) found that nearsighted people were 60 percent more likely to have glaucoma than people with normal vision (not nearsighted). Interestingly, this study also found an association between farsightedness (hyperopia) and ocular hypertension (elevated IOP without glaucoma damage). Researchers were surprised by this finding because farsightedness is usually just associated with increased risk for primary angle-closure glaucoma (see chapter 4 for description), and not ocular hypertension.

## SIGNIFICANT EYE INJURY

Trauma to the eye from accidents and injury increases the risk for glaucoma. But trauma is not the only potential cause of eye injury. Any eye surgery—cataract surgery, retinal surgery, vitrectomy, corneal surgery—should be considered an eye injury or trauma that can lead to glaucoma. In fact, glaucoma after corneal transplant surgery is one of the most difficult glaucomas to control.

An exception to the postsurgical risk factor is the vision-correcting LASIK surgery, which has not been shown to increase the incidence of glaucoma. However, it is important to know that *the LASIK procedure does result in a thinning of the cornea.* And since IOP is currently and routinely measured using instruments (the Goldmann tonometer) that rely on certain assumptions related to the cornea and its thickness, *eyes that have had LASIK show lower IOP readings because of the thinning of the cornea.* For instance, the IOP may measure 21 mm Hg after LASIK with Goldmann tonometry, but will actually be higher than that—perhaps as high as 25 or 30 mm Hg. A formula to calculate that exact IOP number has not yet been determined but is being researched. Many are looking forward to that result. Central corneal thickness

(CCT) and its associated risks are discussed more fully in chapter 5.

## LONG-TERM USE OF CORTISONE OR STEROIDS

Cortisone and steroids include eyedrops or ophthalmic ointments and inhaled steroids, like nasal sprays, as well as oral, IV, and injected medications such as prednisone and solumedrol. The important variables to consider with this risk factor are dosage, route of administration, and duration of medication use. The likelihood of developing elevated IOP from steroids varies with each of these factors. Topical ophthalmic steroids (medications put *on top* of the skin) are more likely to raise IOP than systemic steroids (medication taken *into* the body). Injection of steroids directly into or onto the eye is very risky because these steroids often have a prolonged action. Fortunately, not everyone develops increased IOP as a result of taking steroid medications. Steroid-induced glaucoma is discussed in chapter 4.

## HIGH BLOOD PRESSURE

Patients with high blood pressure have an increased risk of developing glaucoma. However, as I stated in chapter 1, blood pressure and intraocular pressure vary independently. Blood pressure control does not indicate that your IOP is being controlled. Similarly, if you are under a great deal of stress and your blood pressure rises, it doesn't necessarily follow that your IOP will also rise. Blood pressure and eye pressure are independent of one another.

## LOW BLOOD PRESSURE (ESPECIALLY WITH A SUDDEN DROP AT NIGHT, DURING SLEEP)

We now understand that for some people, or in some forms of glaucoma, there is a strong link between glaucoma and poor (reduced) blood flow to the optic nerve. Patients who are taking medication to control high blood pressure may actually have their blood pressures dropping to very low levels during the hours they are sleeping. This reduces the amount of blood flow to the eye and optic nerve and may compromise the optic nerve. Therefore, patients with any progressive form of glaucoma (that is, patients in whom the visual field test and/or optic nerve appearance are worsening despite controlled IOP) need to make sure their blood pressure is not dropping to very low levels while they sleep—or at any time during the day or night. This is a good example of why the eye has to be considered as a part of the entire body—not just an organ alone, in isolation. Your ophthalmologist needs to know about all your medical conditions and which medications you are taking. Your eye doctor must work with all your other doctors to make sure that everyone is in sync.

## THIN CORNEA

A thin (or thinner-than-average) cornea has recently been associated with an increased likelihood of developing glaucoma in certain groups of people. An important study of people with ocular hypertension (OHT—elevated IOP without glaucoma damage to the optic nerve or visual field) revealed that people with OHT who had thinner central corneas were more likely to develop glaucoma. This important study, called the Ocular Hypertension Treatment Study (OHTS) is discussed at length in chapter 12.

It is also important to understand that central corneal thickness—in addition to being a risk factor for glaucoma when thin—relates to inaccuracies in measuring IOP. For individuals with thin CCT (thinner-than-average central corneal thickness), IOP measurements tend to be underestimated, possibly leading them (and their physicians) to miss a very significant risk factor of elevated IOP. On the other hand, measurements of IOP tend to be overestimated in people with thick corneas (thick CCT). Recently, the measurement of CCT has become an integral part of evaluating an individual's glaucoma risk and in determining optimal glaucoma management.

## PLAYING THE TRUMPET, FRENCH HORN, OBOE, OR PICCOLO

The trumpet, French horn, oboe, and piccolo are high-resistance wind instruments. Some small clinical studies suggest that playing such instruments may be associated with an IOP elevation dependent on the force of the blowing and a possible visual field deterioration related to the cumulative number of hours spent playing.

This is a very minor risk, and few people should refrain from playing these instruments because they fear glaucoma damage. But if you do play one of these instruments, it is wise to make your eye doctor aware of it.

## WEARING A TIGHT NECKTIE

A 2003 clinical study by Dr. C. Teng and colleagues showed that wearing a tight necktie can result in an elevation of IOP. This occurs, presumably, because the tight necktie exerts pressure on the jugular vein, thus causing elevated venous pressure and elevated episcleral venous pressure (EVP), which in turn elevates IOP. The increase in IOP that results from a tight necktie may also increase the risk of developing glaucomatous changes in the optic nerve. More study of this potential risk factor is needed.

*Chapter 4*

# Types of Glaucoma

In this chapter, I will discuss many different forms of glaucoma. I will also briefly describe the best methods of treating each of them. A more complete and detailed explanation of these treatments—medication, laser surgery, traditional surgery, and even future advances—will be found in chapters 6 through 9 and 14. But since each kind of glaucoma may involve its own unique form of treatment, this chapter would not be complete without a brief mention of the treatment options. (The sections on the less-common glaucomas may not contain much treatment information.) First, however, I will discuss factors that are common to all types of glaucoma.

## THE COMMON THREAD AMONG ALL FORMS OF GLAUCOMA: GLAUCOMATOUS OPTIC NEUROPATHY

As you no doubt realize by now, *glaucoma* is a term that refers to many different disorders. There are many glaucomas. Each of these shares a common endpoint: a specific type of damage to the optic nerve. This damage is formally called *glaucomatous optic neuropathy.* Glaucomatous optic neuropathy can vary in its severity and appearance, presenting itself in a number of ways. It may present itself as localized defects or erosions of the saucer portion of the optic nerve head (the neuroretinal rim). There may be localized loss of nerve fibers in one specific area that can be preceded by a small, localized hemorrhage at the edge of the optic nerve head. There could be an overall enlargement of the optic cup in a diffuse fashion. Or the doctor might notice deepening of the cup, displacement of the vessels on the surface of the optic nerve head, development of asymmetry of the cup-to-disc ratios between the two eyes, or increased pale coloration (pallor) of the optic nerve head (this is related to a greatly enlarged cup). Small hemorrhages may also be noticed within the thin layer of nerve fibers adjacent to the optic nerve head. Figure 12a illustrates the optic nerve head and visual field of someone with end-stage glaucoma.

You will notice that I have not mentioned elevated intraocular pressure (IOP) as a common factor in all glaucomas. That is because not all forms of glaucoma are associated with elevated IOP. However, as I discussed in chapter 1, Glaucoma Myths, elevated IOP is a significant risk factor for glaucoma. In general, IOP of 10 to 21 mm Hg (millimeters of mercury) is considered normal, and IOP above 21 mm Hg is considered elevated. But some people develop damage to the optic nerve at normal levels of IOP (normal-tension glaucoma, or NTG). On the other hand, other people can tolerate high IOP levels without affecting nerve cells (ocular hypertension, or OHT).

## PRIMARY OPEN-ANGLE GLAUCOMA (POAG)

This is the most common form of glaucoma in the United States, accounting for approximately two-thirds of all cases.

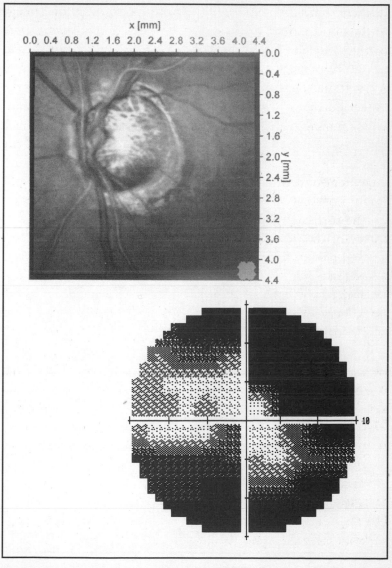

**Figure 12a.** Advanced, end-stage glaucoma: The cup-to-disc ratio is greater than 0.9 (over 90 percent cupping of the disc). There is nasal displacement of the blood vessels. The visual field shows extensive damage. The dark areas indicate where sight has been lost: This patient has only a small island of vision remaining.

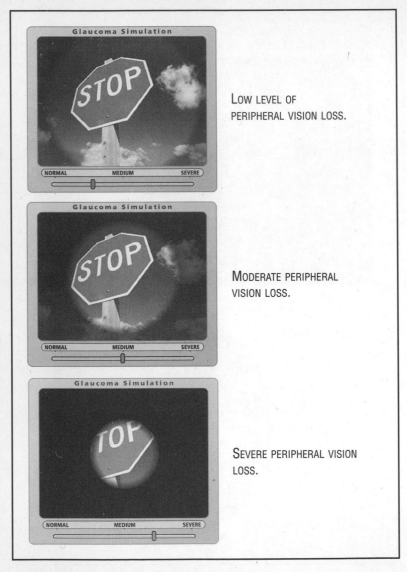

**Figure 12b.** How POAG affects peripheral vision.
(Courtesy of the Xalatan Web site, Pharmacia Ophthalmology)

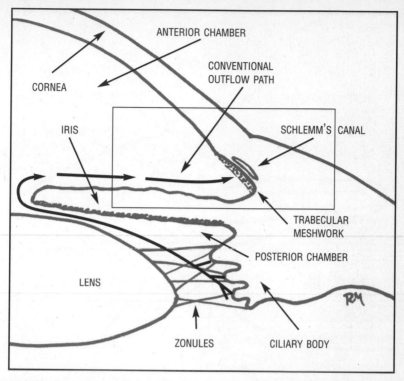

**Figure 13a.** The normal angle (showing the conventional outflow pathway).

Typically, in POAG, there is a gradual rise in IOP rather than a sudden, rapid onset of elevation. There is no apparent cause or initiating event, and there is no outward sign that IOP elevation is occurring. The cornea does not swell. There is no blurred vision. There is no pain. There are no noticeable symptoms. Without symptoms, a person with undetected, untreated glaucoma does not realize what is happening until vision is permanently affected. Usually, peripheral vision is affected first and central vision is affected later in the course of the disease (figure 12b).

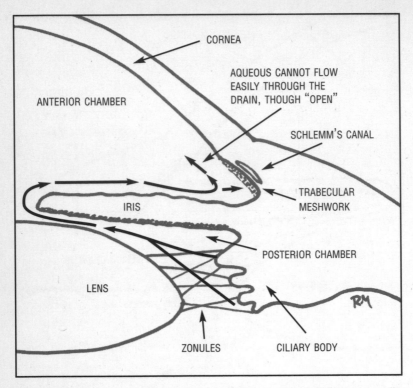

**Figure 13b**. Open-angle glaucoma: Aqueous cannot flow normally through the trabecular meshwork, resulting in an elevation of IOP.

## What Is POAG?

There are many different forms of open-angle glaucoma. In fact, they should probably be called "the open-angle glaucomas." You will see that many of the glaucomas described in this chapter are open-angle glaucomas. Basically, the name is derived from the fact that the angle formed by the intersection of the iris and the cornea is "open" (figure 13a). (Remember, *angle* refers to the structures within the area where the iris meets the cornea. The term also refers to the specific way in which the iris meets the cornea, forming an angle that is wide open, or narrow, or closed.)

In examining the angle and the trabecular meshwork in a patient with POAG, it would appear that the aqueous would flow freely through. The trabecular meshwork may appear to be perfectly normal. However, the aqueous cannot properly escape because of a resistance to flow within the eye's drainage system (trabecular meshwork and related structures).

### Who Gets POAG?

Primary open-angle glaucoma is present in at least 2 percent of the over-forty-year-old population worldwide. It is difficult to obtain an accurate statistic because the definition of what constitutes open-angle glaucoma is not always consistent among studies. What we do know is that the incidence of glaucoma is increasing rapidly as the world's population ages.

Why does the incidence of this type of glaucoma increase with age? Does something happen to the eye's drainage system as we get older? Yes, indeed. There is a narrowing of the spaces through which aqueous flows out of the eye. In addition, there is an age-related reduction in the size of Schlemm's canal. These (and other) factors may contribute to the association between the increased risk of POAG and aging.

The onset of POAG is typically in those over age forty-five. There are usually no symptoms, and damage to the eye may take many years to occur. POAG *can* occur in patients under forty-five, but when it does, the signs and symptoms may vary from the norm.

Younger patients with POAG may experience blurred vision or halos around lights. This can be a sign that the eye pressure is significantly elevated and has become elevated over a relatively brief period of time. Remember, though, that this is an exception! There are usually no symptoms associated with POAG until the disease is quite advanced.

### How Is POAG Diagnosed?

The diagnosis of POAG is often made during a routine eye exam. Although I will discuss the classic tests for glaucoma later in this book, typically, with POAG, the diagnosis is made by evaluating three key variables: measuring the IOP (tonometry), assessing the appearance of the optic nerve, and visual field testing. In classic POAG, the IOP is elevated, the optic nerve shows cupping, and the visual field shows areas of vision loss. As with all forms of glaucoma, the patient may not become aware of visual field changes until a significant amount of vision has been permanently lost.

### How Is POAG Treated?

The treatment for POAG is to lower the IOP. In the United States, this is initially accomplished most often by medication (usually eyedrops). If medical therapy fails, laser trabeculoplasty is usually considered next. This is a laser procedure in which laser energy is applied to the trabecular meshwork to improve aqueous outflow and lower IOP. If laser trabeculoplasty fails, glaucoma filtration surgery performed in the operating room may be required. In some instances (and more often outside the U.S.), laser or surgery may be chosen as the initial treatment for POAG, not medication. (This trend for *earlier* laser treatment for POAG is increasing rapidly among American glaucoma specialists as the safety and effectiveness of the newest laser, selective laser trabeculoplasty, is being demonstrated. You will learn more about SLT in chapter 14.)

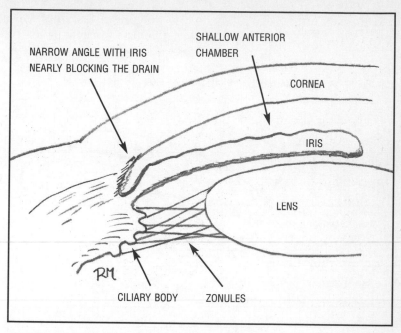

NARROW ANGLE WITH IRIS
NEARLY BLOCKING THE DRAIN

SHALLOW ANTERIOR
CHAMBER

CORNEA

IRIS

LENS

RM

CILIARY BODY    ZONULES

**Figure 14.** The narrow angle: The anterior chamber is shallow, with the iris lying closer than normal to the cornea. Aqueous is able to reach the trabecular meshwork (drain) through this narrow inlet (where the iris meets the cornea).

## PRIMARY ANGLE-CLOSURE GLAUCOMA (PACG)

In primary angle-closure glaucoma, the angle (in a susceptible person) formed by the intersection of the iris and the cornea is *smaller* than normal. This is called a narrow angle (figure 14).

The angle in a normal, healthy eye is at least forty degrees. The angle in an eye that is predisposed to primary angle-closure glaucoma is usually twenty degrees or less. In this form of glaucoma, the trabecular meshwork may work normally, but the peripheral iris blocks the flow of aqueous out of the anterior chamber by preventing its access to the meshwork. The result is elevated IOP. When the angle is open, the IOP is usually

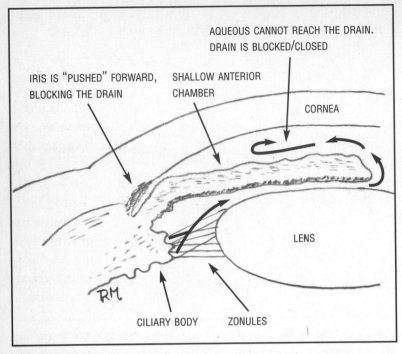

**Figure 15.** Angle-closure glaucoma: Note that the iris is "pushed" forward, blocking the drain.

normal; when the angle is closed (figure 15) and only a portion of the eye's drainage system is allowing aqueous to flow out, IOP rises proportionately.

Anything that dilates the pupil can bring on an attack of angle-closure glaucoma in a susceptible eye. Possible precipitating factors include eyedrops used to dilate the pupil during an eye exam; dim light; stress; oral medications such as anticholinergics, antihistamines, antinausea medications, or cold medications; and botulism toxin. (It is interesting and important to note that when the package insert for a medication warns that the medication should be "avoided if you have glaucoma," it usually means that the medication tends to dilate the pupil and could precipitate an attack of angle-closure glaucoma in a person with a susceptible, narrowed angle.)

## Who Gets PACG?

PACG occurs most often in farsighted people—particularly farsighted women in late middle age. In fact, it occurs in women three to four times more frequently than in men. The fact that the prevalence increases with age may be related to a thickening and forward movement of the lens that naturally occurs with age.

In most populations, PACG is seen less often than POAG. This is true in the United States. In some populations, however, PACG is *more* common than POAG. Epidemiologic studies have shown that PACG predominates among Alaskans, Greenland Inuit, and Asians. PACG is uncommon among African Americans, while POAG is much more common in that population than in Caucasians.

A family history of PACG adds to the risk of developing this type of glaucoma. Among first-degree relatives (parents, siblings), the risk of PACG is 2 to 5 percent. Another factor that increases risk is a thin, flaccid iris. When a patient has this type of iris, it can more easily bow forward and close the drain. This is more apt to occur in the elderly and people with blue irides.

Those people who are most predisposed to angle-closure glaucoma have very distinct eyes. These eyes have a shallow anterior chamber, a narrow angle (the most distinguishing characteristic), and possibly a thick and more anteriorly positioned lens.

There are three main types of PACG: acute ACG; intermittent (or subacute) ACG; and chronic ACG.

### Acute Angle-Closure Glaucoma (AACG)

In acute angle-closure glaucoma, the angle between the iris and the cornea closes suddenly and there is a rapid, large rise in IOP (figure 16a). This may occur in darkened rooms such as movie theaters, or during periods of high stress—both of which cause the pupil to dilate and the angle to narrow or close. For obvious reasons, attacks usually occur during the evening. They also occur more often in autumn and winter. (There are *more* attacks of AACG when there are *fewer* hours of sunlight!) Medications that dilate the pupil can also precipitate attacks. People with narrow anterior chamber angles are at risk for attacks of primary acute angle-closure glaucoma.

Unlike POAG, acute angle-closure glaucoma is associated with a sudden onset of distinct symptoms: blurred vision, eye pain, halos around lights, headache, nausea, vomiting, and mid-dilated (partially dilated) pupils.

When the IOP rises by a large amount over a brief period of time, as in AACG, the cornea becomes swollen with fluid. Termed corneal edema, this causes blurred vision and the appearance of halos around lights. The eyelids may swell. The whites of the eye appear red. The edematous cornea may look as if it is steamy or may resemble ground glass. The anterior chamber can be so shallow and the cornea can be so cloudy during these attacks that it is often difficult for the doctor to see inside the affected eye. On examination, if the cornea is clear enough to allow a view, the doctor sees that the angle is closed. Early in the course of the attack, the optic nerve head may appear hyperemic (increased amount of blood with engorged blood vessels). A severe and prolonged attack leads to the optic nerve head appearing pale and cupped.

Acute angle-closure glaucoma is a *medical emergency* that, if not treated immediately, can result in permanent vision loss. Medications are used first to lower the IOP and allow the swollen, edematous (fluid-filled), and cloudy cornea to clear. The doctor may use a gonioscopy mirrored lens to press on and indent the cornea to help break the attack (open the angle). Miotic drops (which constrict the pupil) such as pilo-

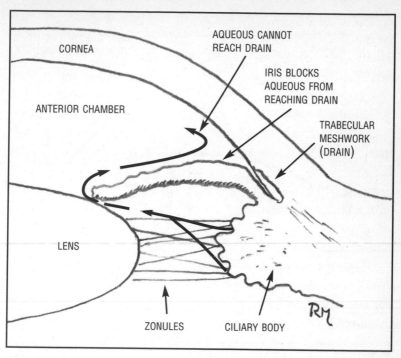

**Figure 16a.** Angle-closure glaucoma attack *before* laser peripheral Iridotomy (LPI): Note that the peripheral iris is blocking the trabecular meshwork. Aqueous is unable to exit the eye, causing IOP to rise significantly.

carpine, in a low percentage such as 1 or 2 percent, are given. Usually pilocarpine is given one drop every five minutes for four doses. This will make the pupil become small and pull the iris away from the angle, thus breaking the attack. Oral glaucoma medications (such as acetazolamide or methazolamide) are often used in combination with eyedrops to help lower the IOP as quickly as possible.

When the cornea becomes sufficiently clear, the doctor will perform a laser peripheral iridotomy (LPI). This is a procedure in which laser energy is used to make an opening through the

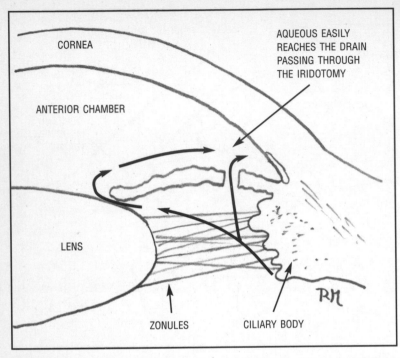

**Figure 16b.** Angle-closure glaucoma attack *after* laser peripheral irido-tomy (LPI): The peripheral iris no longer blocks the trabecular meshwork, and aqueous is able to flow through the iridotomy. The anterior chamber deepens, and the iris resumes a more normal position.

iris, allowing aqueous to move easily from the posterior chamber into the anterior chamber (figure 16b). In some cases, laser gonioplasty (laser to the peripheral iris) may help pull the iris away from the angle and break the attack. Gonioplasty is a procedure in which laser energy is applied to the surface of the peripheral iris—the portion of the iris that lies closest to the eye's drain (trabecular meshwork). The laser spots cause the iris tissue to contract and pull away from the drain. As the iris pulls away from the drain, the drain is reopened and aqueous is able to enter it, thus breaking the glaucoma attack.

The dilemma facing the doctor when this condition is encountered is that this condition should be treated with a laser peripheral iridotomy as soon as possible in order to lower the IOP. However, the cornea is usually swollen with fluid and cloudy during an attack, so the doctor may not see well enough to perform the procedure. Laser light cannot pass easily through an edematous cornea to perform the much-needed iridotomy. Hopefully, the doctor's maneuvers to clear the cornea and lower the IOP will succeed and the laser surgery can be performed before the optic nerve is damaged and vision loss occurs. *Remember: This is an emergency situation, and time is of the essence!*

Once the doctor has performed the laser peripheral iridotomy, he or she will carefully check the angle for the presence of scar tissue that can form during an angle-closure attack. This scar tissue is called peripheral anterior synechiae (PAS). PAS represents scar tissue that seals the iris onto and often *over* the trabecular meshwork, blocking the flow of aqueous in that area. If PAS areas are present after the attack, the doctor may want to treat these with an argon or YAG laser to further restore flow of aqueous into and through the trabecular meshwork. Clearly, the best prognosis is associated with attacks that have not led to the development of PAS.

Recurrent episodes of acute angle closure may be quite damaging to the eye. They can lead to permanent PAS formation and permanent closure of the angle.

## A CRUCIAL FACT

Laser peripheral iridotomy—a brief, painless procedure—should be performed as a preventive measure in the *healthy* (unaffected) eye of people who have had attacks of acute angle-closure glaucoma. Half of all individuals who have had an attack of acute angle-closure glaucoma in one eye will go on to have an attack in the other eye within five years. Because the effects of an attack can be so devastating and vision threatening, preventive LPI is definitely indicated. Once created, the iridotomy's openness (patency) is permanent in almost all instances. The opening in the iris cannot heal itself closed. For most patients who have an LPI, the procedure does not have to be repeated. (Note: Some physicians call this procedure a peripheral iridectomy because a small portion of the iris is being "removed." Others call it a peripheral iridotomy because a small opening, or hole, is created within the iris. Throughout my training, my colleagues and I have used the term *iridotomy* because it was believed to be more accurate. Both terms are technically correct. In this text, I will use the term *iridotomy* for this laser procedure.)

---

### Primary Intermittent or Subacute Angle-Closure Glaucoma (ACG)

Patients with this type of ACG have mild, brief attacks of angle closure that spontaneously resolve—perhaps by the pupil constricting when moving into the light, or by sleep. Unfortunately, these mild, brief attacks of ACG tend to recur.

Symptoms of primary intermittent or subacute angle-closure glaucoma include an ache in the eye, slightly blurred vision, or halos around lights. The treatment is laser peripheral iridotomy.

### Primary Chronic Angle-Closure Glaucoma (PCACG)

Individuals with this type of glaucoma have a progressive closure of the angle that often leads to sustained IOP elevation.

Initially, there may be attacks of angle closure without PAS (scar tissue formation between the iris and the cornea). Later on in PCACG, as more angle-closure attacks occur, PAS areas are formed. On examination of eyes with primary chronic ACG, the IOP is elevated and the eye appears uninflamed (quiet). There is no corneal swelling because the IOP has been rising gradually, rather than suddenly. The optic nerve exam reveals cupping. The visual field exam is abnormal and is consistent with the optic nerve exam.

Treatment includes laser peripheral iridotomy. If the IOP stays elevated, glaucoma medications are given. If these steps fail to reduce the IOP enough, laser trabeculoplasty (laser procedure where laser energy is applied to the eye's drain to improve drainage) to the open portion of the angle or filtration surgery (trabeculectomy) should be considered (see chapters 7 and 8).

## Other Variants on Angle-Closure Glaucoma

• *Combined-mechanism angle-closure glaucoma:* This is a disorder in which patients have both open-angle glaucoma and closed-angle glaucoma.

• *Plateau iris syndrome:* In this uncommon condition, an iridotomy fails to prevent the development of angle closure. In plateau iris configuration (figure 17), the peripheral iris is bent sharply forward so that the iris lies extremely close to the trabecular meshwork. However, the central iris plane is flat. Plateau iris configuration is caused by ciliary processes or ciliary cysts that push the peripheral iris forward onto the eye's drainage system (trabecular meshwork), potentially causing angle closure. This primarily affects young people (women more than men) in their thirties through fifties. Treatment to prevent angle closure in plateau iris configuration includes laser peripheral iridotomy. Once an LPI has been performed, IOP is

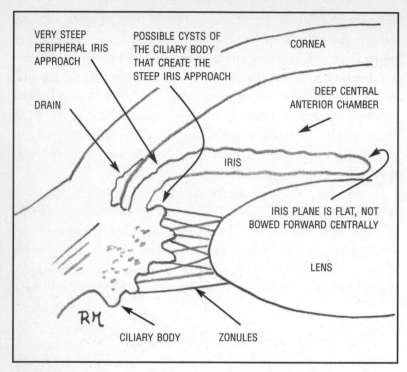

**Figure 17.** Plateau iris configuration: The peripheral iris has an extremely steep approach at the angle. The anterior chamber is deep centrally. The iris has a flat, plateau-like configuration in combination with a very steep, narrowed approach at the angle. The iris is not bowed forward centrally. High frequency ultrasound may show cysts of the ciliary body.

remeasured and the doctor performs a gonioscopy (view the angle through a gonioscopy lens). This allows the doctor to visualize the angle and trabecular meshwork. In plateau iris syndrome, gonioscopy shows that the peripheral iris still lies extremely close to the drain (trabecular meshwork), despite the LPI. The doctor should also perform a mydriatic provacative test. To do this, the doctor uses medication to dilate the patient's eye. Then he or she views the angle with a mirrored lens.

If the angle appears very narrowed or closed after dilation using eyedrops, despite a patent (open) LPI, a diagnosis of plateau iris syndrome is made. Initial treatment for plateau iris syndrome includes medications, such as pilocarpine, to pull the peripheral iris away from the angle. If this fails, argon laser gonioplasty may be performed to contract the peripheral iris so that it pulls away from the angle.

## NORMAL-TENSION GLAUCOMA (NTG)

Normal-tension glaucoma can also be referred to as normal-pressure glaucoma. NTG—another form of glaucoma in which the angle is open—is often difficult to diagnose and can easily be overlooked in a routine eye exam.

In normal-tension glaucoma, the IOP is *not* elevated. Unlike other forms of glaucoma, the level of IOP often does *not* correlate with the amount of optic nerve damage or the visual field abnormality. However, despite a lack of IOP elevation in NTG, the optic nerve does become cupped and the visual field test shows loss of vision (figure 18). This form of glaucoma is now recognized as occurring more commonly than once thought. NTG may account for as many as one-third to one-half of all cases of open-angle glaucoma. *(Ethnicity matters a great deal. A study of Japanese people with glaucoma found that 78 percent had IOP levels below 21 mm Hg!)* Whether NTG is a variant on POAG or a completely different form of glaucoma is being debated heavily among glaucoma specialists.

In most forms of glaucoma, patients tend to lose peripheral vision first. However, in normal-tension glaucoma, the initial visual field defect is typically near the center of the field, near central vision (near "fixation"). This tendency to develop near-fixation visual field defects makes normal-tension glaucoma especially frightening. In addition, NTG tends to be a very aggressive and progressive form of glaucoma.

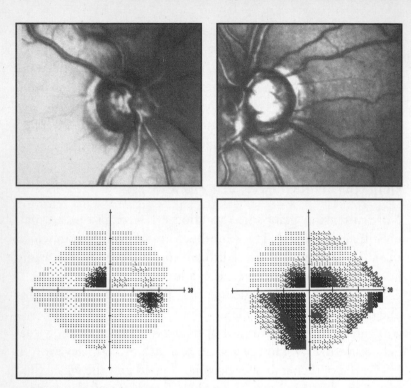

**Figure 18.** Normal-tension glaucoma: The disc on the left shows a patient who has newly diagnosed NTG, with thinning of the lower portion of the rim of the disc. This corresponds to a visual field abnormality in the area near fixation (paracentral visual field defect). The disc on the right shows a patient with NTG with advanced cupping and a large paracentral visual field abnormality.

## How Is NTG Diagnosed?

The following guidelines can help diagnose normal-tension glaucoma:

- IOPs less than or equal to 21 mm Hg.
- Open angles, as seen during gonioscopic exam (an exam

in which a mirrored lens is placed on the eye so that the angle can be viewed by your doctor).

- The optic nerve shows typical glaucomatous change with cupping and rim loss.
- No secondary cause for the optic nerve changes (no precipitating disease or trauma).
- Visual field changes are consistent with the optic nerve changes. (Often, in NTG, the visual field defects are not as peripheral, as they are in other forms of glaucoma. Instead, they are near the center of vision. Doctors term this "near fixation.")
- Progression of glaucomatous damage over time, despite normal IOP levels.

With this definition, as many as one-third to one-half of all cases of open-angle glaucoma can be classified as normal-tension glaucoma. It is often difficult to delineate clear lines between POAG and NTG.

## What Causes NTG?

Doctors are actively seeking the causes of NTG. It may be an autoimmune neuropathy. (Autoimmune diseases are those in which the body's immune system attacks itself and specific organs or tissue of the body. Neuropathy is a disease or disorder that attacks the nervous system.)

Here is some of the evidence that NTG may be autoimmune in nature:

- Approximately one-third (30 percent) of patients *with NTG* have been documented to have some form of a known autoimmune disease, as compared to 8 percent of individuals *without NTG*.
- Patients with NTG often test positive for auto-antibodies

(proteins produced as part of an immune response "to self"), which are most typically seen in people with auto-immune disease.

Despite these compelling findings, the role of autoimmune disease in NTG remains unproven. Research in the area is on-going.

There may be a vascular cause for NTG. Optic disc hemor-rhages (small hemorrhages on the surface or edge of the optic nerve head) are more common in normal-tension glaucoma patients than in POAG.

Some experts believe that a vascular cause for NTG relates strongly to poor blood flow to the optic nerve. It has been re-ported by many glaucoma doctors that poor blood flow to the optic nerve may result from nocturnal hypotension (blood pressure that's too low at night and/or during sleep). Systemic nocturnal hypotension is a clue that a person with NTG has a poorly regulated vascular system. There is further evidence to support a poorly regulated vascular system in NTG. Specifi-cally, NTG patients often have migraine headaches, Raynaud's syndrome, and small hemorrhages in the optic nerve head.

In NTG, as in other forms of glaucoma, a genetic inheri-tance is likely. I will discuss the role of genetics in glaucoma in chapter 15.

### How Is NTG Diagnosed?

Your ophthalmologist should always take a medical history the first time he or she sees you. An especially detailed medical history is critical if your doctor suspects normal-tension glau-coma, which has been associated with such health problems as Raynaud's syndrome (in which the extremities become so cold that they may actually turn blue), elevated cholesterol, mi-graine, autoimmune disorders, and low blood pressure.

Other possible diagnoses that your doctor might consider before determining that you have normal-tension glaucoma include:

- Primary open-angle glaucoma (POAG) in which elevated IOP was not detected, but is present nonetheless. This would include people with POAG in whom there have been large IOP variations during the day (diurnal variations) or night (nocturnal), and the IOP was always recorded during the times of normal IOP.

- Low central corneal thickness (CCT) in a person with POAG. IOP is measured as low or normal (not elevated) in individuals with thin CCT.

- Intermittent elevations (or spikes) of IOP that are actually related to another form of glaucoma. Some forms of glaucoma, such as angle-closure or inflammatory glaucoma, cause *intermittent*—rather than *constant*—elevations of IOP. In these cases, damage to the optic nerve would occur when IOP is elevated. Depending on when the IOP is measured, the doctor could miss seeing the periods of IOP elevation and misdiagnose the patient as suffering from NTG.

- It is possible that past episodes of elevated IOP may have created the optic nerve damage that is currently being investigated.

- The doctor should ask about a history of severe blood loss or hypotension (low blood pressure), because compromised blood flow to the optic nerve could have caused the optic nerve damage.

- The patient should be asked which medications are being taken, since certain drugs—oral beta-blockers in particular—may lower IOP.

In diagnosing NTG, the doctor usually considers other uncommon diagnoses that can mimic it, such as congenital anomalies, compressive lesions (such as tumors) of the optic nerve or chiasm (for example, a mass that presses on the optic nerve or part of the eye's neurologic connection to the brain).

A systemic workup (general physical exam plus blood tests—and possibly a neurologic evaluation) may be considered in rare cases of suspected normal-tension glaucoma in patients who have some or all of the following characteristics:

- Age less than 60.
- Reduced vision without obvious cause.
- An abnormal visual field that is not characteristic of glaucoma.
- Optic nerve pallor (pale coloration).
- Visual field defects and optic nerve appearance that do not correlate.
- Marked asymmetry of the optic nerve heads between the two eyes.
- Rapid progression of visual field loss.

There are some specific tests that should be considered in cases of suspected normal-tension glaucoma. One such test is the *diurnal curve*, which maps out the IOP over time, throughout the day and sometimes at night. A diurnal curve records the levels of IOP over time and looks for any IOP spikes that could lead to damage to the optic nerve. Central corneal thickness should be measured to be certain that the IOP level measurement is accurate and not underestimating the IOP.

## How Is NTG Treated?

Normal-tension glaucoma is a particularly difficult form of glaucoma to treat and control. It tends to be a progressive disease—worsening despite treatment. Patients with a history of migraine headache or optic disc hemorrhage are at greater risk for damage and progression. Women are also at higher risk for damage and progression than men. For patients with this condition, careful and frequent monitoring of the appearance of the optic nerve head and the visual field are crucial.

Since nocturnal hypotension is a significant risk factor in NTG, it is important that the eye doctor work closely with the internist. To confirm nocturnal hypotension, a patient's internist may obtain blood pressure readings throughout the day, evening, and night. If medications for hypertension are causing the drops in blood pressure, these should be changed. If not, the internist may consider using salt tablet supplements or medicine (e.g., Florinef) to bring the blood pressure level to an acceptable range.

Our understanding of normal-tension glaucoma is incomplete. However, a study performed by the Collaborative Normal-Tension Glaucoma Group has shown that despite the fact that IOP levels are normal in this condition, lowering the IOP *is protective* in many patients. Often the pressure has to be maintained at levels that are below normal: less than 10, where normal range is 10 to 21 and elevated IOP is greater than 21. Reducing the IOP by 30 percent is considered by most glaucoma specialists to be protective, lowering the chance of glaucoma progression.

How does your doctor lower the IOP by 30 percent or more? Initially, eyedrops can be used to reduce IOP. Currently, it is not known if any of today's medications provide neuroprotection (protection of the optic nerve and/or retinal ganglion cells) or improve ocular blood flow. If medical treatment fails to lower IOP sufficiently, laser trabeculoplasty (argon laser trabeculoplasty—ALT, or selective laser trabeculoplasty—SLT) should be considered. Often filtering surgery is required to lower the IOP to the required low level.

People with normal-tension glaucoma usually need to see their doctors more frequently than do those with POAG. The frequency of eye exams depends on many factors, including level of IOP, the health of the optic nerve, how well medications are being tolerated, and whether or not the doctor is changing the drug regimen. If you have NTG, your doctor may have you perform a visual field test and have your optic nerve examined as often as every three or four months. But remember, the frequency of doctor visits will depend on your unique needs. Clearly, successful management of NTG requires diligent monitoring by the eye doctor *and* strict compliance on the part of the patient!

## PIGMENTARY GLAUCOMA

Pigmentary glaucoma is a form of glaucoma associated with abnormal distribution of pigment within the anterior chamber and the deposition of this liberated pigment onto various structures within the eye.

The pigment being referred to in this condition originates from the iris. This pigment is liberated from the iris surface or, more accurately, from the posterior (back) surface of the iris. Once liberated, this pigment floats within the anterior chamber and deposits itself on such structures of the eye as the cornea, the trabecular meshwork, the front surface of the iris, and the lens. The cells that line the trabecular meshwork beams are phagocytic, which means that their purpose is to eat and remove debris and pigment. The phagocytes become overloaded by all the pigment and die. Thus the trabecular beams can no longer rid themselves of pigment and debris. The result is an increased resistance to outflow. Aqueous is less able to escape from the eye, causing IOP to rise.

## Who Gets Pigmentary Glaucoma?

It is possible to have pigment dispersion without glaucoma, but often they go hand in hand. Typically, *pigment dispersion syndrome* (without glaucoma) is found in younger people—age twenty through forty-five—but it can also occur in older people. *Pigmentary glaucoma* occurs more often in men than in women. Women with pigmentary glaucoma tend to be older (forty to fifty) than men with this disorder. Whites are more commonly affected than blacks and Asians. Nearsightedness is often seen with this condition.

Nearsightedness (myopia) is a very important risk factor in pigmentary glaucoma. The greater the degree of nearsightedness, the younger the age in which glaucoma damage may be seen. Vigorous exercising (especially high-impact exercise) in susceptible individuals (not everyone) or having the pupils dilated may liberate pigment and cause spikes in IOP, blurred vision, and/or halos. (See chapter 11 for more on exercise and pigmentary glaucoma.)

## What Causes Pigmentary Glaucoma?

What is the cause of this abnormal liberation of pigment? Pigment may be liberated from the posterior (back) surface of the iris because of an inherited susceptibility to pigment liberation. (As mentioned, I will further discuss genetics and advances in glaucoma genetic research in chapter 15.) Pigment liberation may also occur in some people because of the natural shape of their irides, which causes rubbing of the iris against the lens zonules. In these patients, there is often a very deep (deeper-than-normal) anterior chamber and a significant posterior bowing of the peripheral iris. (The iris bows backward, toward the lens and zonules.) This leads to friction between the back, pigmented surface of the iris and the lens zonules. The friction leads to the release of pigment. In addition, friction might occur between the lens and iris during blinking and when the eye focuses on close objects.

### How Is Pigment Dispersion Syndrome or Pigmentary Glaucoma Diagnosed?

On exam, the doctor may notice that the dispersion of pigment occurs in both eyes (bilateral) but is asymmetric (not equal). This is very common. On examination of the cornea, the doctor may notice a vertical, spindle-shaped deposit of pigment on the innermost surface of the cornea. This is called a Krukenberg Spindle. The iris may also show radial slitlike defects in the midperiphery of the iris. These defects are often best seen through a technique called transillumination. In transillumination, the light from the slit lamp shines into the pupil directly, and the doctor observes the way in which the light bounces back out of the eye through these abnormal slits in the iris. The lens surfaces may also show deposits of pigment, and a ring of pigment may be seen on the posterior peripheral surface of the lens.

Here is some good news: As a person with pigmentary glaucoma gets older, the amount of iris pigment released often decreases and the condition may improve. The patient may experience better IOP control, fewer IOP spikes, and a gradual lessening of the amount of pigment visible within the eye's drain. In addition, presbyopia (loss of accommodation) reduces the contact between the posterior surface of the iris and the lens zonules, slowing the release of pigment.

## How Is Pigmentary Glaucoma Treated?

Pigmentary glaucoma is treated by lowering the IOP. As in POAG, eyedrops are generally used first. If IOP control is not achieved, laser trabeculoplasty or filter surgery may be needed.

Some glaucoma specialists use an eyedrop (pilocarpine) to help flatten the iris and prevent the iris from rubbing against the lens and zonules. Pilocarpine, unfortunately, is often not well tolerated. It can blur and dim vision, accelerate cataract formation, or predispose a person to retinal detachment. Alternatively, laser peripheral iridotomy may be used to cause the posteriorly bowed iris to assume a more flattened shape. This flattened shape of the iris leads to less friction between the iris and the lens zonules. However, the effectiveness of LPI is controversial and debated among glaucoma specialists.

## NEOVASCULAR GLAUCOMA (NVG)

Neovascular glaucoma is a secondary glaucoma (it develops as a result of another medical condition or event such as diabetes or eye trauma). In this condition, there is abnormal, vascularized tissue in the angle that blocks the drain (trabecular meshwork). This abnormal tissue pulls the iris into the angle, blocking the trabecular meshwork and causing the IOP to rise. This type of glaucoma usually occurs after an ischemic retinal event (an event in which the retinal blood supply is compromised).

When the retinal blood supply is significantly compromised, a substance called vasoproliferative factor (or angiogenic factor) is released from the retina. This factor stimulates the growth of new blood vessels within the anterior chamber. The new vessel growth is called neovascularization of the iris (NVI). As this progresses, a neovascular membrane can grow into the angle. With shrinkage or contraction of this membrane, the iris is pulled into the angle, blocking the drain. PAS may form as well.

### What Causes NVG?

Ischemic central retinal vein occlusion (CRVO—a blockage in the central retinal vein) is a common cause of NVI, producing more than one-third of all cases of NVI. Fifty percent or more of the retina must be ischemic (inflow of blood is obstructed) for NVI to occur. The more blockage of blood flow within the retina, the greater the risk for neovascular glaucoma. If only a small branch vessel of the retina is blocked, NVI does not occur.

Most cases of neovascular glaucoma occur within one hundred days after a central retinal vein occlusion. That is why this type of glaucoma is often referred to as the "hundred-day glaucoma."

People with diabetes are at greater risk of developing neovascular glaucoma. Diabetic retinopathy (abnormal vascular changes—such as leakage and new vessel growth—in the retina related to diabetes) is responsible for one out of three cases of NVG. Neovascular glaucoma has been found to occur in 2 percent of all diabetics and 21 percent of patients with proliferative diabetic retinopathy (more advanced stage of diabetic retinopathy in which new, abnormal blood vessels develop in the retina).

Carotid artery occlusive disease (blockage of either of the two main arteries that travel up the neck on either side and supply blood to the head) is the third most common cause of neovascular glaucoma, occurring in 13 percent of all cases. Other causes of neovascular glaucoma include central retinal artery occlusion (blockage of the artery that supplies blood to the retina) and ocular tumors (such as malignant melanoma or retinoblastoma).

## How Is NVG Diagnosed?

In neovascular glaucoma, the IOP is high and the cornea is often swollen, edematous (swollen with fluid, or fluid-filled), and cloudy. There is inflammation inside the anterior chamber, and often blood from the abnormal, leaky new vessels is present. On examination, the doctor frequently sees new blood vessels growing on the iris—especially at the margin of the pupil. The doctor looking at the angle with a gonioscopy (mirrored) lens sees that there are many adhesions between the iris and the angle. Over time, there is a zippering effect in which the angle progressively gets "zipped closed" as more and more adhesions form.

## How Is NVG Treated?

The doctor's goals in the treatment of neovascular glaucoma are pain relief, reduction of inflammation, preservation of vision, and preservation of the eye.

In this form of glaucoma, eyedrops are used but are often unable to control the IOP. Miotic medications (like pilocarpine) are avoided since they increase inflammation by increasing the permeability of the blood aqueous barrier. Cycloplegic drops (such as Cyclogyl and atropine) often reduce pain and improve uveoscleral (the nonconventional outflow path for aqueous, discussed in chapter 3) outflow. Topical steroids are used to reduce inflammation and pain.

The main, initial therapy for neovascular glaucoma is pan retinal photocoagulation (PRP). By lasering the retina, the release of vasoproliferative factor is decreased. Scar tissue formation within the angle (drain) is not reversed with PRP, but progression of scar tissue formation is usually stopped.

Another treatment that helps prevent the release of vasoproliferative factor is cryotherapy (treatment with extreme cold) of the retina. Cryotherapy is especially useful in cases when the doctor cannot easily see the retina. (Remember that your doctor must be able to visualize the retina to effectively laser it.)

Glaucoma shunt procedures (valves) are often used by surgeons to control the IOP in NVG. Filtration surgery (trabeculectomy) is often chosen when there is good visual potential in the patient. Cyclodestructive procedures (procedures that reduce IOP by damaging the ciliary body and causing a reduction in the amount of aqueous produced) are usually reserved for people in whom other procedures have failed to control the IOP—or when there is very poor potential for useful eyesight. (Doctors term this *poor visual potential.*)

For patients who have lost their sight but have severe pain as a result of neovascular glaucoma, injection of alcohol behind the eye may produce temporary or permanent pain relief. Surgical removal of a blind, painful eye may be required if all else fails.

## EXFOLIATION SYNDROME AND EXFOLIATIVE GLAUCOMA

Exfoliation syndrome is a systemic disorder. This means that it is a disease that affects the entire body and not just the eye. Exfoliation syndrome causes clinical signs within the eye and affects the eye in specific ways, often involving glaucoma.

In exfoliation syndrome, the eye produces a white, fluffy material within its anterior segment. This material is also found in the conjunctiva, the extraocular muscles (muscles outside the eye), the sheath (covering) of the optic nerve, and the skin.

## Who Gets Exfoliation Syndrome?

Exfoliation syndrome is most common in whites and is uncommon in African Americans. Its prevalence increases with age. It affects women more than men. However, if a man has exfoliation syndrome, he is more likely to develop glaucoma. A study reported in the 2003 *Journal of Glaucoma* found the incidence of exfoliation syndrome to be 26 people per 100,000 population, and the incidence of exfoliative glaucoma to be 10 people per 100,000 population. This syndrome is also strongly associated with cataract formation. Furthermore, in this type of glaucoma, the IOP often fluctuates greatly.

*Exfoliative glaucoma* is associated with open angles. It is believed that the exfoliative material blocks or damages the trabecular meshwork and causes IOP to rise. Other possible causes of elevated IOP in this condition include the deposition of pigment within the trabecular meshwork, which causes blockage, or the creation of abnormal blood vessels in the iris.

Nevertheless, some exfoliation syndrome patients may have narrow anterior chamber angles. This narrowing of the angle could be related to the weakening of zonules that is typically seen with this condition. Although exfoliation syndrome is most commonly associated with open-angle glaucoma, it *can* be associated with angle-closure glaucoma.

## How Is Exfoliation Syndrome Diagnosed?

What does the doctor see when looking inside the eye of someone with exfoliation syndrome? Typically, there is a fluffy whitish material deposited on the front surface of the lens in a specific pattern. There is a central area of lightly deposited whitish material, a peripheral zone with more heavily deposited fluffy material, and a clear zone separating the two.

Exfoliative material can also be found on the cornea, the

front surface of the vitreous, and the posterior capsule after cataract surgery. Zonules may have deposits of exfoliative material on them as well. The iris might show transillumination defects, especially in the area near the pupil. The area of the iris near the pupil often appears thin, and clinicians describe it as appearing to be moth-eaten. As a result, the pupil dilates poorly. Dilating the pupil often leads to pigment release and elevation of IOP. Pigment is seen deposited on the front surface of the iris and in the angle. In fact, pigment within the angle can sometimes be the first visible sign of exfoliation syndrome. (Although this may sound similar to pigmentary glaucoma in some ways, it is actually quite distinct. These two glaucomas are *not* easily confused by doctors.)

Another unique finding the doctor looks for in this syndrome is pigment that is deposited on the surface of the angle, anterior to Schwalbe's Line. This "line" of pigment is called Sampolesi's Line, which is very common in patients with exfoliation syndrome and is considered to be diagnostic of exfoliation syndrome.

### How Is Exfoliative Glaucoma Treated?

The treatments for exfoliative glaucoma are similar to those for primary open-angle glaucoma and usually begin with eyedrops. However, patients with exfoliative glaucoma usually respond *less well* to medications than patients with POAG. (An important fact!)

Patients with exfoliative glaucoma have an initial response to argon laser trabeculoplasty that is better than in patients with POAG. But often, there is a post-laser IOP elevation that is significant. (For this reason, doctors usually monitor the post-laser IOP closely in patients with exfoliative glaucoma.) If medical and laser therapy fail, surgical intervention with a filtering procedure (trabeculectomy) is recommended.

As mentioned earlier, people with exfoliative glaucoma often have cataracts. The surgical technique used to remove the cataract in the presence of exfoliative glaucoma is technically demanding for a number of reasons, which I'll explain in more detail in chapter 9. To minimize the difficulties associated with this cataract surgery, it is best to perform the cataract removal *earlier rather than later*. When the cataract surgery is not de-layed and done promptly, the lens is more easily emulsified by ultrasound (phacoemulsification—see chapter 9), creating less stress on the zonules. *Operating earlier makes for safer surgery when treating a cataract in someone with exfoliation.*

## CORTICOSTEROID GLAUCOMA

This is a form of open-angle glaucoma that is associated with topical (eyedrops and ointments), periocular (injection onto, near, or behind the eyeball), and, less commonly, systemic (oral, inhaled, intravenous, injected) corticosteroid usage or exposure.

Why would someone be on steroids in the first place? Steroids are used to reduce inflammation. Steroid eyedrops are commonly prescribed by doctors to reduce inflammation after surgery or to treat inflammation inside the eye (iritis, vitritis) or inflammation on the surface of the eye (conjunctivitis, ker-atitis). Steroid ointments are often prescribed for inflamma-tions of the ocular surface or lids (blepharitis). Periocular steroid injections may be used to treat inflammations of the retina or vitreous, or inflammations of the tissue around the eyeball. Systemic steroids such as prednisone are often used to treat asthma, rheumatoid arthritis, and autoimmune diseases.

Corticosteroid glaucoma can greatly resemble POAG, ex-cept that the IOP tends to be quite high and of a more sudden onset. Generally, steroids must be used for at least two weeks before the eye pressure is elevated—more commonly, this is seen after three to six weeks. However, IOP elevations have been reported as early as the first week of steroid usage.

The effect of steroids on IOP depends on whether or not the patient has glaucoma. Individuals with POAG are far more susceptible to steroid-related elevations in IOP than individuals without glaucoma.

### Who Gets Corticosteroid Glaucoma?

Risk factors for developing corticosteroid glaucoma include primary open-angle glaucoma, a family history of first-degree relatives (parents, siblings) with primary open-angle glaucoma, nearsightedness, diabetes, rheumatoid arthritis or other connective tissue disorders, and eyes with traumatic angle recession (trauma to the trabecular meshwork that ultimately leads to a blockage of drainage and reduced outflow of aqueous). Most important, though, are the *strength*, *frequency*, *duration*, and *type* of steroid used. In steroid-induced glaucoma, the IOP increase is usually short term, but the longer the exposure to the steroid, the greater the chance that the IOP will stay elevated after the steroid has been discontinued.

### What Causes the IOP to Rise in Corticosteroid Glaucoma?

IOP appears to rise because of an increased resistance to aqueous outflow. There are a number of possible causes for this increased resistance. Prolonged steroid exposure may lead to an abnormal accumulation of mucopolysaccharides that cause reduced flow of aqueous through the drain. Steroids may also alter the collagen elastin and fibronectin that form the filter through which the aqueous must flow. Poor flow of aqueous through the drain leads to an elevation of IOP. Additionally, steroids may slow down the process by which the trabecular meshwork cells dispose of waste particles, resulting in a clogging of the trabecular meshwork and poor drainage of aqueous. Finally, steroids may cause a reduced production of prostaglandins, substances that may alter aqueous outflow. Since IOP elevation may be more immediate when systemic steroids are involved, the cause of the related IOP rise may have more to do with an overproduction of aqueous than a problem with outflow.

### How Is Corticosteroid Glaucoma Treated?

Treatment of corticosteroid glaucoma involves discontinuing the steroids or shifting to a weaker formula. If the IOP stays elevated and threatens to create optic nerve damage, filtration surgery could be required. Laser trabeculoplasty does not work well with corticosteroid glaucoma.

The bottom line: *Use corticosteroids cautiously.* IOP must be monitored closely in *all* patients who use steroids, whether they are used topically or systemically. In addition, patients using steroids must be educated about their risk for elevated IOP and the need for regular examination and IOP measurement. *Do you know people who are using steroids? Steroid inhalants for asthma? Prednisone for arthritis? These folks need to have their eyes checked!*

## GLAUCOMA ASSOCIATED WITH ELEVATED EPISCLERAL VENOUS PRESSURE (EVP)

The episcleral veins are located in the connective tissue between the sclera and the conjunctiva. EVP is the pressure in the veins that drain aqueous fluid after it passes through the trabecular meshwork. The normal drainage pathway of aqueous is seen in the flow chart on page 74.

anterior chamber

trabecular meshwork

Schlemm's canal

collector channels

episcleral veins

The fluid moves in this direction because of a pressure gradient (difference in pressure) between the IOP and EVP. So if EVP is elevated, there is less of a pressure gradient, and thus the drive to move aqueous out of the eye (and lower the IOP) is reduced . . . and IOP becomes elevated.

Elevated EVP may cause glaucoma through another mechanism. EVP can be elevated because of poor flow through the vortex veins (the veins that allow blood to exit the eye). In this case, congestion causes the choroid to become edematous and swollen. This choroidal swelling pushes the iris and lens forward, leading to secondary angle-closure glaucoma.

Normal episcleral venous pressure (EVP) is 8 to 12 mm Hg. There are several possible causes of elevated EVP. One is Sturge-Weber syndrome, which I will discuss in the next section. Other causes include vascular obstructions (blood clots within the vessels), tumors behind the eye (retrobulbar tumors), or the protrusion of the eyeball due to thyroid disorders. Playing high-resistance wind instruments such as the trumpet, French horn, oboe, and piccolo can cause elevated EVP and can result in an elevation of IOP and glaucoma.

Wearing tightly tied neckties could raise IOP by a similar mechanism.

### How Is Glaucoma Associated with Elevated EVP Diagnosed?

When the doctor looks in the eye of a person with elevated EVP, he or she will note that the blood vessels beneath the conjunctiva are very engorged, swollen, and enlarged. There are no signs of inflammation to explain these congested blood vessels. A simple test by the doctor will show that the affected blood vessels are not on the surface of the conjunctiva (superficial); these blood vessels do not constrict when the doctor applies drops such as phenylephrine. Superficial veins would whiten and disappear in response to the drops. But engorged veins that lie below the surface of the conjunctiva do not respond in this fashion.

The eye exam would reveal that the anterior chamber angle is open. Gonioscopy might show blood in Schlemm's canal. The IOP may be elevated to the mid-20s to mid-30s. These findings can be unilateral (one eye) or bilateral (both eyes).

If the elevated EVP has been long standing, there is often angle-closure glaucoma because the iris and lens have been pushed forward due to the congestion.

### How Is Glaucoma Associated with Elevated EVP Treated?

The treatment for this kind of glaucoma is specific to the cause of the elevated EVP. Drops that suppress the production of aqueous are helpful. But medicines alone may not be enough to lower the IOP. Glaucoma filtering surgery may help, but there can be serious complications such as a buildup of fluid in the choroid (choroidal effusion) and intraocular

hemorrhage. A posterior sclerostomy can be performed to reduce the buildup of fluid. This is a surgical procedure in which
a small opening is made in the back part of the sclera. A small
window is cut out of the sclera in the back half of the eye. Its
purpose is to allow fluid, which would normally be trapped in
the choroid, to escape the eye.

## IRIDOCORNEAL ENDOTHELIAL SYNDROME (ICE SYNDROME)

This syndrome represents a group of diseases, each having various degrees of the following: abnormalities of the innermost
layer of the cornea with a buildup of fluid within the cornea,
anterior chamber angle abnormalities, defects in the iris, and
*secondary angle-closure glaucoma.*

There are three variants of ICE syndrome. Yet each of the
three types shares the following characteristics:

- They almost always occur only in one eye, but the other
  eye may have some abnormalities on the innermost part
  of the cornea.
- The onset is during early to middle adult life.
- Women are affected more often than men.
- There are abnormalities of the iris such as atrophy, hole
  formation, and an irregular pupil.
- Fifty percent of patients with ICE develop secondary
  glaucoma.
- Reduced vision and pain associated with ICE correspond
  to secondary glaucoma and related corneal swelling.
- The angle shows many PAS.
- A glasslike (semiclear) membrane may spread from the
  inner layers of the peripheral cornea over the angle and
  onto the outside surface of the iris. The outflow of aqueous is blocked by this membrane, which covers the tra-

becular meshwork, or by the PAS that may form within the angle.

The three different types of ICE syndrome are most easily distinguished from one another based on the appearance of the iris. These variants are progressive iris Atrophy, Chandler's syndrome, and Cogan-Reese syndrome.

### Progressive Iris Atrophy

This form of ICE syndrome is characterized by the formation of holes in the iris. The iris is very thin and full of irregular holes. Clinicians often describe the iris as appearing to be moth-eaten. The pupil becomes decentered (called correctopia), and the shape of the pupil becomes irregular and often pearlike. Corneal changes are minimal with this form of the syndrome.

### Chandler's Syndrome

This form of ICE syndrome is more common than progressive iris atrophy. A classic finding is that the cornea fills with fluid even if the IOP level is normal. The corneal swelling creates pain, blurry vision, and halos around lights. The endothelial surface has a hammered appearance. There is only mild atrophy of the iris. The pupil is minimally distorted, and few PAS exist.

### Cogan-Reese Syndrome

The key findings in this form of ICE syndrome are pigmented nodules on the surface of the iris. In other words, it looks as if the iris is covered with numerous, tiny, pigmented bumps or elevations (nodules). Microscopic examination of

these nodules shows portions of normal iris surrounded by abnormal cellular membranes.

What causes Cogan-Reese syndrome? Some believe it is
caused by a virus. Others believe there may be a basic defect in
the cornea, which leads to the creation of the cellular membrane.

### How Is ICE Syndrome Treated?

Elevated IOP related to this syndrome can be treated with
aqueous suppressants and hypotensive lipid eyedrops. Miotic
eyedrops such as pilocarpine should be avoided. Filtering surgery is often needed and is usually successful. However, the
filtering surgery may fail later—perhaps even years later—because the cellular membrane found in these patients continues
to grow, blocking the filter drainage site. Shunts rarely work in
these cases. Corneal transplant may also be required because of
the chronic corneal swelling.

## GLAUCOMATOCYCLITIC CRISIS (POSNER-SCHLOSSMAN SYNDROME)

This disorder is characterized by unilateral (relating to one eye)
attacks of glaucoma. The attacks, which recur and are associated with mild inflammation, are associated with extreme elevations of IOP. The IOP level may reach 40–60 mm Hg.

This syndrome usually affects people between the ages of
twenty and fifty. The cause is unknown but may be related to
the immune system.

During an attack, symptoms are extremely mild in relation
to the extreme elevations of IOP. The patient complains of
slight discomfort, blurred vision, and halos around lights. On
exam, the doctor sees mild inflammation and a swelling of the
cornea. The eye may be slightly red, and the pupil may be con-

stricted. There may be collections of inflammatory cells on the inner corneal surface. These collections of inflammatory cells are called keratic precipitates (KP). The anterior chamber angle remains open without any PAS. The rise in IOP may be related to inflammation in the trabecular meshwork (called trabeculitis). There may also be increased aqueous production.

An attack lasts hours to weeks. Between attacks, the affected eye has normal IOP. Usually there is a normal visual field and optic nerve. However, if attacks are repetitive and of long duration, glaucoma damage results.

This condition is usually self-limited, meaning that the attacks can end by themselves. Topical steroids reduce inflammation and help lower IOP by improving trabecular outflow. Indomethacin and other cyclo-oxygenase inhibitors may also help lower IOP. Glaucoma medications are often given to reduce IOP, although miotics should be avoided. Filtration surgery may be needed if glaucoma damage occurs.

The doctor usually follows patients with this syndrome very carefully because they are more likely than nonaffected individuals to have a coexisting primary open-angle glaucoma.

## FUCHS HETEROCHROMIC IRIDOCYCLITIS

This disorder is characterized by mild, unilateral chronic inflammation of the ciliary body (cyclitis) associated with the two eyes being a different color (termed heterochromia iridis), cataract, and sometimes glaucoma. It is bilateral (relating to both eyes) in only about 10 percent of patients. It affects men and women equally. The disorder usually occurs between the ages of thirty and forty, and its cause is unknown. There are usually no symptoms—no pain, irritation, redness, or light sensitivity. Reduced night vision may occur as the only complaint.

Upon examination, the doctor observes a very mild, chronic

inflammation. Inflammatory deposits on the inner surface of the cornea are common. These are typically fine and colorless, unlike the case of other forms of uveitis. In about 20 percent of cases, small nodules can be seen on the iris near the pupillary border.

The iris of the involved eye can be darker or lighter than the uninvolved eye. Sometimes the iris develops a thinned, irregular appearance that is described as appearing to be moth-eaten. When this occurs, the affected eye may look darker because pigmentation on the back surface of the iris is exposed and is quite dark in color.

Chronic inflammation in the eye can lead to a specific form of cataract often seen in this disease called a posterior subcapsular cataract (PSC). Cataract surgery improves vision but can be complicated postoperatively by inflammation and glaucoma. After surgery, vision may be reduced somewhat because of pigment deposits that can form on the new lens that has been implanted.

Approximately 25 percent of patients with this condition develop glaucoma. The risk of glaucoma is increased if the condition is long standing, bilateral, or the patient is black. The glaucoma involves an open rather than a closed angle.

Steroids are not helpful and may worsen the cataract and glaucoma. In fact, controlling the inflammation has little influence on the glaucoma. Eyedrops should be used to control the elevated IOP. Miotics and argon laser trabeculoplasty should be avoided. If medications fail, glaucoma filtration surgery is usually performed.

# GLAUCOMA ASSOCIATED WITH LENS DISORDERS

## Phacolytic Glaucoma

The term *phacolytic* refers to the breaking down of the lens (*phaco* means "lens"). In phacolytic glaucoma, a very advanced and swollen cataract (the eye's natural crystalline lens when it is opacified and no longer clear) leaks protein into the anterior chamber, creating inflammation. The so-called scavenger cells, or macrophages, travel to the anterior chamber to remove this protein. However, the macrophages also block the outflow channels of the trabecular meshwork, causing an elevation in IOP.

This type of glaucoma is usually unilateral (occurring in one eye). It is associated with pain and blurred vision. Upon examination, the doctor will notice swelling of the cornea and inflammatory cells in the anterior chamber. The anterior chamber will contain tiny particles of whitish material both floating in the aqueous and deposited on the front surface of the lens.

To accurately diagnose this type of glaucoma, the doctor may choose to perform a paracentesis, which involves making a small opening into the cornea and removing some fluid from the anterior chamber. The fluid can then be examined for evidence of lens proteins and inflammatory cells. However, the diagnosis is typically made through a clinical exam alone.

This condition is initially treated with eyedrops and oral medications to reduce IOP. Miotics should not be used because they often increase inflammation. In fact, medication to reduce inflammation is required. Cycloplegics, such as Cyclogyl or atropine, are also required to dilate the pupil. Why dilate the pupil? Dilating the pupil is analogous to putting your arm into a sling after an injury. Just as the sling keeps the elbow from moving around as it heals, dilating the pupil (the "moving part" inside your eye) prevents the pupil from opening and closing repeatedly. This allows the inflammation to resolve more quickly.

Once medications are instituted to reduce inflammation and IOP, the definitive treatment is removal of the cataract.

### Phacomorphic Glaucoma

This is a type of glaucoma associated with swelling of a cataractous lens but without leakage from the lens. The lens is swollen and enlarged, and the thickening of the lens pushes the iris forward. The iris blocks the drainage channels, and the IOP rises. Aqueous builds up in the posterior chamber, causing the iris to bow forward. This is called iris bombé (pronounced *bom-BAY*).

As a cataract develops, it often becomes thicker, just as a tree trunk gets thicker with age. As the lens thickens, pupillary block increases. Medications such as pilocarpine or other miotics can aggravate the situation and increase pupillary block, increasing the risk of angle closure.

The treatments for phacomorphic glaucoma are eyedrops and oral medications to reduce the IOP. Laser peripheral iridotomy is usually indicated to prevent angle closure. Once these measures have been taken, cataract removal is indicated.

### Ectopia Lentis

In this condition, the lens of the eye has been displaced from its usual position. If the lens is only partially displaced, it is called subluxation, because it is being held partially in place by the zonules. When the lens is completely displaced from its usual position this is called dislocation.

The symptoms associated with this condition usually include blurred vision, inability to accommodate (focus things nearby), and double vision out of one eye.

On examination, the doctor will notice that the iris moves, shakes, and quivers easily. This phenomenon is called iridodenesis. The doctor may also notice that the lens moves, shakes, and quivers easily. This is called phacodenesis. The margin of the lens may be seen, especially when the pupil is dilated.

Glaucoma can result from ectopia lentis in multiple ways. It may occur when the lens moves forward into the anterior chamber or backward into the posterior chamber. Or glaucoma may develop as a result of significant inflammation. The treatment for this condition includes removal of the dislocated lens.

There are a few inherited conditions or disorders that might cause ectopia lentis. These include Marfan syndrome, homocystinuria, Ehlers-Danlos syndrome, Weill-Marchesani syndrome, Stickler syndrome, hyperlysinemia, megalocornea, and others. Lens dislocation can also be acquired, such as through trauma, surgery, exfoliation syndrome, high myopia, intraocular tumors, hypermature cataract, and uveitis.

## GLAUCOMA FOLLOWING CATARACT SURGERY

Cataract surgery involves removing the eye's natural (but clouded) lens and replacing it with a clear implant. During the surgery, viscoelastic materials are used to stabilize and protect the eye and allow easy insertion of the implant. The most common viscoelastic materials include Healon, Amvisc, Viscoat, Ocucoat, and Healon 5. After the surgery has been completed, all of the viscoelastic material is usually removed. However, if it is not completely removed, the material blocks the trabecular meshwork, resulting in a temporarily elevated IOP as this material slowly exits the eye over several days. It is also possible for blood and inflammatory and/or pigment debris to block the trabecular meshwork and raise IOP after cataract surgery. All of the above would account for causes of *early* post-cataract IOP elevation.

*Late* postoperative glaucoma may be caused by steroids (this usually begins after two to three weeks) or chronic inflammation. There is also a syndrome called the UGH syndrome, which stands for uveitis (inflammation inside the eye) glaucoma (elevated IOP) hyphema (blood in the anterior chamber of the eye). The UGH syndrome is most common with anterior chamber intraocular lens implants (AC IOLs). Unlike a posterior chamber IOL (PC IOL), which sits within the capsular bag from which the cataract is removed, the anterior chamber IOL sits in the anterior chamber. An anterior chamber IOL is in direct contact with the trabecular meshwork, and inflammation is not uncommon.

Late postoperative glaucoma may also result from retained lens material, pigment dispersion, or ghost cells (described elsewhere in this section). Glaucoma may also occur following a YAG laser capsulotomy procedure, which is performed to resolve blurry vision in people who have had cataract surgery. This kind of blurry vision is common and occurs in up to 50 percent of patients undergoing cataract surgery, but glaucoma associated with this procedure is uncommon. The doctor should wait a minimum of three months after cataract surgery before YAG capsulotomy is performed.

Glaucoma can also be related to wound leakage or iris incarceration within the incision after cataract surgery. In this type of glaucoma, a membrane begins to grow and block the trabecular meshwork (termed epithelial downgrowth). The prognosis with this form of glaucoma is very poor, because it is difficult to treat. Medications are unable to sufficiently lower the IOP. Filtration surgery may be an initial success but frequently fails as this abnormal membrane continues to grow. Fortunately, this type of glaucoma is extremely rare.

Angle-closure glaucoma can also follow cataract surgery.

This occurs most commonly with the use of an anterior chamber intraocular lens, especially if there is postoperative inflammation.

## GLAUCOMA RELATED TO SURGERY

### Aqueous Misdirection Syndrome

Also called malignant glaucoma (unrelated to cancer) or ciliary block glaucoma, this is typically a syndrome that occurs after glaucoma or cataract surgery in which there is shallowing or flattening of the anterior chamber and elevation of IOP related to angle closure, despite the presence of an open (patent) iridectomy or iridotomy. Once the anterior chamber shallows, there is a forward shift in the lens and iris. The flow of aqueous from the posterior chamber into the anterior chamber becomes blocked. Aqueous redirects itself into the vitreous. The flow of aqueous directly into the vitreous pushes the iris and lens forward so dramatically that it may completely flatten the anterior chamber.

Aqueous misdirection syndrome is also characterized by a lack of response or worsening of IOP with the use of miotics such as pilocarpine.

This syndrome can occur in patients who have undergone cataract surgery, filtration surgery, or combined cataract and filtration surgery. It also can occur following surgical iridectomy, cyclodialysis, or full-thickness glaucoma procedures (see glossary for descriptions). Its occurrence has also been documented following laser iridotomy, but is rare.

Aqueous misdirection syndrome occurs in 2 to 4 percent of eyes undergoing glaucoma surgery. This is especially true in eyes whose filters naturally allow an excessive amount of aqueous to escape from the anterior chamber, which can cause the anterior chamber to become shallow. Small, hyperopic eyes and eyes with shallow anterior chambers and PAS are predisposed to developing aqueous misdirection syndrome.

Aqueous misdirection syndrome is diagnosed when, upon examination, the doctor notices a shallow or flattened anterior chamber, an elevated IOP, and an open (patent) iridectomy or iridotomy. Initially, the IOP may be normal, but it's *definitely not low*. This is an important point because a shallow or flat anterior chamber with a low IOP indicates overfiltration, wound leak, or both. Ultimately, as more and more aqueous is misdirected into the vitreous, a dramatic elevation in IOP occurs.

*This condition demands immediate medical treatment.*

Miotics are discontinued. Patients are given cycloplegic drops such as atropine 1 percent four times a day. The atropine *temporarily* paralyzes the circular or sphincter muscle of the iris and ciliary body. This allows the iris and lens to resume their original position, thus restoring the normal architecture of the eye. Treatment with atropine may be required for months or years. Aqueous suppression is important, since it will reduce the amount of aqueous that flows into the vitreous cavity. Diamox (acetazolamide) and Neptazane (methazolamide) may be very helpful in the management of this emergency condition.

In treating this condition, the doctor needs to help the aqueous leave the vitreous cavity. This is achieved by making a small opening in the most anterior part of the vitreous (the vitreous that is just behind the lens—called the vitreous face). Once the vitreous face is opened or disrupted (by laser or surgery), aqueous can flow forward into the anterior chamber, restoring the anterior chamber depth and breaking the syndrome. The exact surgical technique will vary depending on whether or not the patient's lens has been surgically removed. If the eye's natural lens has been removed, YAG laser will be sufficient to make the opening in the vitreous face. If the eye's natural lens is still present, surgery in the operating room is needed.

If the anterior chamber angle of the other eye is narrow, a laser peripheral iridotomy should be performed. If the other eye is to undergo glaucoma surgery, the doctor can reduce the chances of having an attack of this particular type of glaucoma by avoiding miotics, avoiding hypotony (low IOP) after surgery, avoiding overfiltration, avoiding wound leaks, and using atropine during and after surgery for one month.

### Glaucoma Following Penetrating Keratoplasty (PK)

The incidence of glaucoma after penetrating keratoplasty— better known as corneal transplant—may be as high as 31 percent. Risk factors include preexisting glaucoma, previous cataract surgery, previous vitrectomy (removal of the vitreous), previous corneal transplant, or a history of eye inflammation. After a corneal transplant, the IOP may fluctuate tremendously and damage the transplant. (The new corneal graft does not do well when there is elevated IOP or when multiple medications are needed to control IOP.)

Glaucoma may occur soon after corneal transplant—or much later. Some causes of glaucoma soon after corneal transplant surgery are related to blood in the vitreous or inflammation of the uvea. After corneal transplant surgery, there may be a lack of support for the trabecular meshwork, which also may be collapsed and unable to allow aqueous to escape normally. Corneal transplant surgery may also alter the angle structures. Inflammation may lead to blockage of the trabecular outflow. If viscoelastic materials are used during PK and are not completely removed by the doctor during surgery, this may cause IOP to rise (significantly, but temporarily).

Later in the course, inflammation and PAS may cause angle closure. Or steroid-induced glaucoma may occur because prolonged use of steroids is often required with this procedure.

Glaucoma following corneal transplant surgery is very diffi-

cult to treat. Medications are tried first, but often fail to sufficiently lower the IOP. Filtration surgery and/or shunts are performed next, but these often fail also. The failure of glaucoma
surgeries in these patients' eyes may be related to inflammation
within the eye after PK.

### Glaucoma After Scleral Buckle (Retinal Detachment Surgery)

In one common type of retinal detachment surgery, a band-
like device called a scleral buckle is placed around the eye. The
pressure on the vortex veins (the large veins that drain the uvea
and exit the eye through the sclera) causes the ciliary body to
become congested. The anterior part of the ciliary body rotates
forward and pushes the iris against the trabecular meshwork.
This blocks the trabecular meshwork and causes IOP to rise.

### Elevated IOP Associated with Silicone Oil

Doctors often use silicone oil to help keep the retina in place
after it has detached. The silicone fills the vitreous cavity to a
great degree, helping repair a large retinal defect or detachment. On some occasions, the eye is overfilled with the silicone, indirectly causing a significant rise in IOP and blockage
of the drain. In other instances, the silicone itself may find a
path into the anterior chamber of the eye and directly block
the trabecular meshwork, leading to glaucoma.

### Glaucoma Following Intraocular Gas Injection

Intraocular gases are used very commonly in vitreoretinal
surgery. The use of these materials is considered a major breakthrough in retinal detachment surgery and was popularized by
doctors working at New York Presbyterian, Cornell Medical

Center. These gases are used to push a detached retina back into its original position and keep it there while the retina heals and reattaches. In this situation, the gas bubble may move toward the front, causing the lens to move forward, creating pupillary block. In addition, the IOP may rise as the gas expands. Treatment can include positioning the patient's head so that the gas does not move forward into the anterior chamber. Also, some of the gas may be removed from the eye, or a gas–fluid exchange may be necessary to restore the eye's normal inflation. Chronic angle-closure glaucoma may result from PAS formation when the anterior chamber remains shallow during periods of significant postoperative inflammation, as is often seen in these types of surgical cases.

## GLAUCOMA ASSOCIATED WITH TRAUMA

In nonpenetrating trauma (such as being hit in the eye by a tennis ball), the iris, ciliary body, trabecular meshwork, and lens zonules can be damaged, leading to glaucoma. An eye hemorrhage may lead to red blood cells that block the trabecular meshwork. In addition, after such a trauma, there may be a decreased outflow related to inflammation, hemorrhage, swelling, or scarring of the trabecular meshwork. Swelling of the lens or uvea can also cause the lens to move forward, resulting in angle closure. Aqueous misdirection syndrome (malignant glaucoma, as discussed earlier) may occur.

### Ghost Cell Glaucoma

This form of glaucoma results from a blockage of the trabecular meshwork secondary to "ghost cells." Such cells are formed when red blood cells from a hemorrhage break down.

The treatment for ghost cell glaucoma includes medications to lower the IOP and/or washout of the anterior chamber.

During anterior chamber washout, ghost cells are removed by repeatedly irrigating the anterior chamber with balanced saline solution. In some cases, however, a vitrectomy may be needed if a large collection of red blood cells is present.

### Hemolytic Glaucoma

This is a form of open-angle glaucoma that occurs within days or weeks after an eye hemorrhage. It differs from ghost cell glaucoma because it involves a blockage of the trabecular meshwork by macrophages filled with hemoglobin and breakdown products from the blood. Upon examination, the doctor sees reddish brown blood cells in the anterior chamber. The trabecular meshwork is covered with a reddish brown pigment. As in ghost cell glaucoma, the treatment is anterior chamber washout to remove the debris and macrophages that clog the drain. In some cases, vitrectomy may be needed to remove vitreous blood as well.

### Angle-Recession Glaucoma

Angle-recession glaucoma occurs in 60 to 90 percent of patients after blunt ocular trauma. In 6 to 20 percent of patients, this type of glaucoma can develop years (or decades) after the trauma occurs.

In this form of glaucoma, blunt trauma (such as being hit in the eye by a ball or fist) causes a tear to occur in the middle of the ciliary body. Scars and adhesions form on the trabecular meshwork, which results in a blockage of outflow of aqueous. A thin membrane may slowly grow over the angle and further block aqueous outflow.

The treatment for angle-recession glaucoma usually includes medications (eyedrops and pills) that reduce aqueous production. (Medications that reduce uveoscleral outflow may actually cause the IOP to rise.) Laser surgery usually does not help. Steroids may cause the IOP to elevate significantly. Filtering surgery (trabeculectomy) has a lower success rate in patients with this condition relative to patients with primary open-angle glaucoma, but should be performed if the IOP cannot be controlled with medicines.

## GLAUCOMA ASSOCIATED WITH SYSTEMIC DISEASES

### Glaucoma Associated with Uveitis (Inflammatory Glaucoma)

Uveitis is a condition in which there is inflammation within the eye. When this inflammation is present, there is usually reduced aqueous production and the IOP becomes lower, not higher. Sometimes, however, the inflammation within the eye affects the trabecular meshwork and causes the trabecular outflow to be abnormally low, possibly allowing the IOP to initially be normal. Once aqueous production returns to its normal levels as the inflammation resolves, the IOP will rise.

Several systemic diseases that cause uveitis can result in glaucoma. The most common of these diseases include sarcoidosis, HLA-B27-associated diseases, rheumatoid arthritis, systemic lupus erythematosus, Sjögren's syndrome, Crohn's disease, ulcerative colitis, syphilis, tuberculosis, and several others.

The inflammation inside the eye can result in permanent scarring or PAS. Scar tissue may also form at the pupiliary border between the iris and the surface of the lens, called posterior synechiae. If extensive posterior synechiae form, this can prevent aqueous from flowing through the pupil. This causes the posterior chamber pressure to elevate and push the iris forward in a bowed manner, causing a closed angle. This bowing forward of the iris is referred to as iris bombé. In order to prevent the formation of scar tissue after surgery, patients are typically treated with anti-inflammatory drugs or steroids in a variety of forms—topical (eyedrops, ointments), injection, or even systemic (oral, intravenous). Occasionally, immuno-suppressive therapy is even warranted in difficult cases. At times, dilating medications may also be required to prevent formation of synechiae.

IOP in uveitis can be normal, low, or high. Typically, uveitis tends to make it more difficult for aqueous to get out through the drain while reducing the amount of aqueous made. Since these forces oppose one another, the IOP may remain low or normal, even though outflow resistance is increased. IOP may also become elevated for several reasons—mainly secondary to increased outflow resistance.

If uveitis becomes more extensive, it can involve other parts of the eye. The inflammatory changes may cause the iris and lens to move forward, and a narrow-angle situation results. A laser peripheral iridotomy may be needed to alleviate the angle closure.

Filtering surgery in uveitic glaucoma patients is very challenging. Failure is common since these eyes are prone to greater inflammation after surgery, increasing the likelihood of scarring. Reducing inflammation *prior* to surgery plays a significant role in surgical success. Shunting procedures may also be indicated, but are at risk of failure for the same reasons.

## AIDS and IOP

In patients with AIDS, the retina can develop serious, vision-threatening infection and inflammation. Inflammation of the retina and choroid can lead to the forward movement of the ciliary body and angle closure. This can occur bilaterally. The treatment for this form of angle-closure glaucoma is to relax the ciliary muscles by using cycloplegic drops such as Cyclogyl or atropine, steroid drops to reduce inflammation, and eyedrops to reduce IOP. Laser peripheral iridoplasty or trabeculectomy could be necessary.

### Inflammatory Open-Angle Glaucoma Associated with Infectious Disease

This form of OAG is specifically related to the inflammation associated with infectious diseases. Primarily, this involves viral infections including herpes simplex, herpes zoster (shingles), rubella, mumps, influenzas, and HIV. It can also be associated with syphilis, leprosy, toxoplasmosis, and onchocerciasis (river blindness).

In this condition, the infectious disease leads to inflammation, creating inflammatory cells. These inflammatory products—including fibrin, leukocytes, and macrophages—can become trapped in the trabecular meshwork, blocking it. The filtering ability of the trabecular meshwork becomes overwhelmed, and IOP rises. The trabecular meshwork itself can also become inflamed. This is called trabeculitis.

Trabeculitis may be responsible for the IOP elevation associated with glaucoma seen in herpes simplex or herpes zoster or recurrent toxoplasmosis. Chemical mediators such as prostaglandins, cytokines, or nitric acid might be released as a result of the infection and lead to IOP elevation. These chemical mediators might increase the inflammatory reaction and aggravate the poor function of the trabecular meshwork, further reducing the outflow and further raising IOP.

## GLAUCOMA ASSOCIATED WITH INTRAOCULAR TUMORS AND DISORDERS OF THE VITREOUS AND RETINA

### Retinal Detachment

Open-angle glaucoma is more common in patients with retinal detachment than in the population in general. This may relate to an association with nearsightedness (myopia), because nearsighted people are more prone to retinal detachment.

Patients who are predisposed to retinal detachment and have glaucoma should avoid miotics such as pilocarpine, since they can increase the risk of retinal detachment. Topical steroids should be used cautiously after retinal detachment surgery because of the possible associated IOP elevation.

### Schwartz's Syndrome

This syndrome is characterized by elevated IOP in patients with untreated, long-standing retinal detachment and iridocyclitis. The elevated IOP could result from reduced outflow related to the iridocyclitis (inflammation of the iris and ciliary body), or pigment becoming trapped within the trabecular meshwork and blocking the outflow. The inflammation and elevated IOP may possibly be resolved with surgical correction of the retinal detachment.

### Glaucoma Associated with Intraocular Tumors

A variety of malignant and benign tumors can be associated with glaucoma. Open-angle glaucoma occurs more commonly in eyes with tumors involving the anterior segment. The trabecular meshwork may become obstructed by tumor cells, blood, blood products, or inflammatory cells that enter the eye because of tumor necrosis (cell death). Some tumors release pigments that can lead to blockage of the drain.

Angle-closure glaucoma is more common with tumors of the posterior segment, including choroidal melanoma and retinoblastoma. Large tumors of the choroid or retina (or long-standing total retinal detachment) may push the lens and iris diaphragm forward and cause angle-closure glaucoma. Furthermore, tumors may result in neovascularization that may also lead to angle closure.

Glaucoma may also arise from the treatment used for a tumor within the eye. Radiation therapy can damage the retina or ciliary body and lead to neovascular glaucoma with angle closure. Steroids can create steroid-induced glaucoma. Inflammation related to tumor therapy can reduce flow through the trabecular meshwork and raise IOP.

To manage these glaucomas, the doctor must first identify the tumor and then identify the mechanism of the glaucoma. Eyedrops are used to lower IOP. Laser peripheral iridotomy is used for narrowed angles or angle closure. Laser retinal therapy (pan retinal photocoagulation) is used to treat retinal ischemia. Pain control is administered if the eye is blind.

## GLAUCOMA IN CHILDREN

Glaucomas in children are rare: These glaucomas are a group of disorders that represent less than *one-tenth of 1 percent* of all glaucoma patients. Vision loss in these types of glaucoma results not just from optic nerve damage but also from damage to the cornea, astigmatism, and other disorders.

Pediatric glaucomas usually fall into two categories: primary glaucomas, which result from an intrinsic problem with the aqueous outflow path and are genetic; and secondary glaucomas, which result from disorders of the body or eye and may or may not be genetic. Both types may be associated with other medical problems.

### Primary Congenital (Infantile) Glaucoma

Primary congenital glaucoma or infantile glaucoma is the most common type of glaucoma in infants. It occurs in 1 out of 10,000 births in Western countries and 1 in 2,500 births in Middle Eastern countries. Nearly 40 percent of cases are present at birth and 85 percent are diagnosed during the first year of life. It is bilateral (both eyes) in 60 to 80 percent of patients and occurs more frequently in males (65 percent of all cases) than females (35 percent).

In primary congenital glaucoma, there is usually a developmental defect of the trabecular meshwork and anterior chamber angle. The pediatrician usually notices clouding and/or enlargement of the cornea. Parents often report that their child has light sensitivity, tearing, and blinking. Primary congenital glaucoma, unlike secondary infantile glaucoma, is not associated with any easily recognizable congenital abnormality of the iris or any other metabolic, inflammatory, or congenital disease.

Primary congenital glaucoma is usually sporadic but might be genetic. The chance of a second child having it is approximately 1 to 3 percent. If two children have the disease, the chance that additional children will have it rises to 25 percent.

On examining a patient with primary congenital glaucoma, the doctor will find an enlarged eye with a corneal diameter that is larger than normal (buphthalmos). This is because in children, elevated IOP can cause the eyeball itself to enlarge, since the sclera is still very flexible and able to stretch.

Furthermore, the optic nerve of an infant responds differently to elevated IOP than does the optic nerve of an adult. For one thing, it can differ in appearance. In adults, glaucoma usually involves a loss of the optic nerve head's rim tissue, especially at the vertical poles (the six and twelve o'clock positions on the optic nerve head). In children, there may be a generalized enlargement of the cup *without loss of the rim.* There is another aspect of how children's eyes respond to high IOP that is unique: When the IOP is normalized, the optic nerve heads of children or infants can return to a normal appearance. *The cupping can be reversible!* This is not true of adults, in whom cupping is irreversible.

The treatment for infantile glaucoma is usually surgical. The surgery of choice is goniotomy; its rate of success is related to the age of the patient at the time of diagnosis and surgery. Another surgical option is trabeculotomy. This is often chosen if the cornea is not clear because of corneal swelling resulting from high IOP. Both of these procedures are discussed thoroughly in chapter 8.

Sadly, primary congenital glaucoma results in blindness in 2 to 15 percent of individuals. Every child with infantile glaucoma needs to be monitored for a lifetime. Not only can there be a later recurrence of glaucoma, but ocular changes related to the congenital defect can have devastating effects on visual development. For instance, irreversible, extreme nearsightedness may result from enlargement of the globe eyeball. Often patients have "lazy eye" (amblyopia) and visual field loss.

Primary infantile glaucoma can occur later in childhood. When that occurs, the disease is called juvenile glaucoma.

### Sturge-Weber Syndrome

Sturge-Weber syndrome is a congenital disorder characterized by a facial birthmark or "port wine stain." This facial birthmark is the result of a collection of capillaries just beneath the skin. The disorder is usually associated with glaucoma, which may be present at birth or develop during childhood, and with other neurologic disorders.

This birthmark can be present at birth and is usually on one side of the face. X-ray studies of the areas above the eye usually reveal intracranial calcification (small areas of calcifications within the brain) on the same side as the affected eye.

Glaucoma occurs in up to 50 percent of cases of Sturge-Weber. It usually occurs when the facial birthmark covers the lid or the conjunctiva. The glaucoma usually develops in infancy and is on the same side as the birthmark; however, it can also develop later in life.

The elevated IOP associated with this form of glaucoma can be caused by the abnormal development of the angle that blocks the flow of aqueous from the eye or by elevated EVP related to other eye problems related to Sturge-Weber.

When the doctor examines a child with Sturge-Weber syndrome, he or she may see a mass of blood vessels on the lid, episclera, conjunctiva, iris, and ciliary body. There may be a diffuse, orangeish mass seen in the back of the eye.

Eyedrops (especially aqueous suppressants and miotics) may be effective in mild cases of this type of glaucoma and are usually tried as first-line therapy. In infants, the trabecular meshwork is usually very abnormal and surgical intervention is required. The surgeries of choice in these infants are goniotomy or trabeculotomy (not trabeculectomy). After age four, filtration surgery (trabeculectomy) is the procedure of choice if medications are unsuccessful. In these filtration surgeries, the risk of severe complications is great.

Complications of surgery include significant expulsive hemorrhage. Retinal detachment may follow surgery as well. Before surgery, oral agents such as Diamox (acetazolamide) or Neptazane (methazolamide) may help prevent these complications from occurring by bringing the IOP to lower or more normal levels before an incision into the eye is made.

During the beginning of the filtering surgery, the doctor

may perform posterior sclerostomies to help avoid choroidal effusion. At the end of surgery, the doctor makes sure that the newly created filter is very tightly sutured. This seemingly simple maneuver (of tightly suturing the filter site) greatly reduces the risk of vision-threatening hemorrhage, which can occur in these eyes during and after surgery.

## GLAUCOMAS ASSOCIATED WITH VITREORETINAL DISORDERS

### Nanophthalmos

This is a condition in which the eye does not undergo normal development and, as a result, has a greatly reduced volume. The eye has a small cornea, a shallow anterior chamber, a narrow angle, and is extremely farsighted. These eyes can develop acute angle-closure glaucoma, typically between the ages of forty and sixty. In addition, these eyes have a very thick sclera that could be the cause of the angle closure. The thickened sclera may partially block the flow of blood from the eye, causing the uvea to become swollen.

### Persistent Hyperplastic Primary Vitreous (PHPV)

In this condition, a membrane forms behind the lens of the eye. The ciliary processes are pulled into this membrane. This is usually a unilateral (one eye only) condition affecting children. The affected eye is small. Cataract can occur. Glaucoma can be caused by angle closure related to cataract or because the membrane behind the lens causes the lens–iris diaphragm to move forward. Surgery involves removing the cataractous lens and performing a vitrectomy to remove the fibrovascular membrane.

### Retinopathy of Prematurity (ROP)

When an infant is born prematurely, retinal and retinal vascular changes occur. Thirty percent of patients with severe ROP develop angle-closure glaucoma. The glaucoma usually develops late in childhood. An eye with severe ROP usually has an abnormal retina, an abnormal membrane that has formed behind the lens, a small cornea, progressive nearsightedness, a clear lens, and a shallow anterior chamber. Angle-closure glaucoma may be related to a large lens or the membrane behind the lens pushing the lens forward.

## FOR MORE SOPHISTICATED INFORMATION

In this chapter I have given you the most vital—but basic—information on each of the major types of glaucoma. Most of this information has been derived from a collection of well-regarded texts for physicians—primarily ophthalmologists, and particularly glaucoma specialists.

If you would like to know more about the different types of glaucoma and are not afraid to tackle a medical text, I highly recommend the following:*

Shields, M. Bruce. *Textbook of Glaucoma, Fourth Edition.* Philadelphia: Lippincott Williams & Wilkins, 2000.

Epstein, David L. *Chandler and Grant's Glaucoma, Fourth Edition.* Baltimore: Lippincott Williams & Wilkins, 1997.

Morrison, John C, M.D., and Irvin P. Pollack, M.D. *Glaucoma Science and Practice.* New York: Theme Medical Publishers, Inc., 2003.

Gross, Ronald L. *Clinical Glaucoma Management.* Philadelphia: WB Saunders Company, 2001.

*A full list of references can be found at the end of this book.

Boyd, Benjamin F., M.D., Maurice Luntz, M.D., and Samuel Boyd, M.D. *Innovations in the Glaucomas: Etiology, Diagnosis and Management.* Panama City: Highlights of Ophthalmology, 2002.

Eid, Tarek M., and George L. Spaeth. *The Glaucomas: Concepts and Fundamentals.* Philadelphia: Lippincott Williams & Wilkins, 2000.

Ritch, Robert, M. Bruce Shields, and Theodore Krupin. *The Glaucomas, Volumes I and II.* St. Louis: CU Mosby Co., 1989.

# Part II

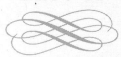

# ESTABLISHED METHODS OF CONTROLLING GLAUCOMA

*Chapter 5*

# Diagnosing and Monitoring Glaucoma

Most forms of glaucoma have no early symptoms. The best way to detect glaucoma is through regular eye exams by your eye doctor.

The three most important factors that your eye doctor carefully determines when making an evaluation for glaucoma are:

1. The appearance of the optic nerve head.
2. The intraocular pressure (IOP).
3. Peripheral vision (visual field test).

All three of these factors must be tested both to detect and to monitor glaucoma.

## GETTING STARTED

An eye exam generally begins with a full medical history and a check of visual acuity—a vision test.

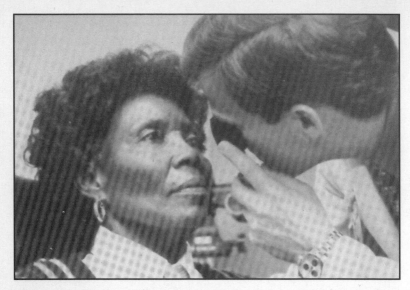

**Figure 19.** Ophthalmoscopy: The doctor is using an ophthalmoscope to examine the optic nerve head (disc). (Photograph by Michael Pollio, Wagern International Photos)

After the vision test follow:

- External exam (looking at the eyelids, eye movement, pupils).
- Slit lamp exam.
- Gonioscopy (looking at the angle).
- Funduscopic exam (ophthalmoscopic exam, looking at the optic nerve head—disc and retina—through an ophthalmoscope). The ophthalmoscope contains a light source and small lenses that allow the doctor to focus on the disc and evaluate its appearance. This is an excellent way to study the optic disc, but it is not a stereoscopic view (figure 19).
- Tonometry (measuring IOP).

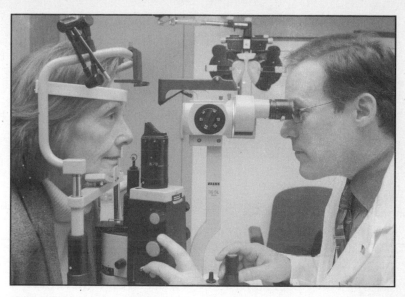

**Figure 20.** The slit lamp exam.

Let's discuss some aspects of the eye exam that relate most directly to an evaluation for glaucoma.

## SLIT LAMP EXAM

If you have had an eye exam, you have probably had the experience of having the ophthalmologist position an instrument in front of you and instruct you to place your chin on the chin rest and your forehead against the headrest (figure 20). This instrument is called a slit lamp. The slit lamp is a microscope with a high-intensity, precisely-focused light source. The term *slit* is used because the beam of light on this device is adjustable from a wide beam to a thin slit of light.

The slit lamp allows the doctor to visualize the structures of the eyes in many different ways. The magnification can be increased or decreased by the turn of a knob. The light source can be varied from dim to bright and from a broad circle of light to a thin slit. A joystick allows the doctor to move the instrument closer to or further away from the patient to optimize the view.

The doctor uses the slit lamp to examine the surface of the eye (conjunctiva, sclera, cornea) as well as the eye's anterior segment (anterior chamber, iris, lens, pupil). With special lenses, the doctor can also examine the back structures of the eye—the vitreous, retina, and optic nerve.

## GONIOSCOPY

Gonioscopy (figure 21a) is a special part of the eye exam that allows your doctor to look into the angle (the area where the iris and cornea meet). It involves placing a special, mirrored contact lens (gonioscopy lens or goniolens) onto the surface of the patient's eye after a numbing drop has been applied. This painless test is performed at the slit lamp. The slit lamp provides illumination and magnification. Gonioscopy is usually performed in a darkened room.

The goniolens allows the doctor to examine the angle (the area where the iris and cornea meet) and determine whether it is open, narrow, or closed, and—if possible—to view the trabecular meshwork (figure 21b).

The smallest of the mirrors is used to view the finest details of the angle. The doctor may be trying to answer some or all of these questions: Is the angle open? Closed? Narrow? Are there peripheral anterior synechiae (PAS), scar tissue or adhesions? Is there a heavy deposition of pigment in the angle? Does the opening that the doctor made surgically during a trabeculectomy appear to be open from the inside?

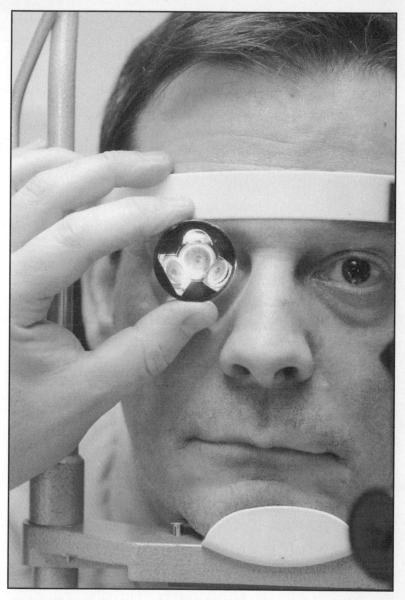

**Figure 21a.** Gonioscopy: A mirrored lens—in this case a three-mirrored lens—is used to view the angle of the eye.

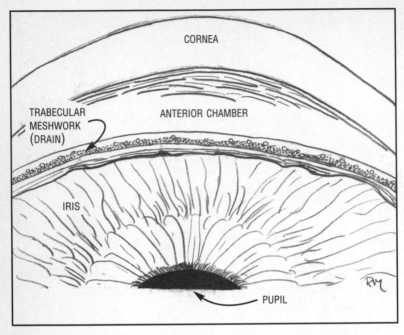

**Figure 21b.** Gonioscopy: The doctor's view. This illustration shows a normal, open angle.

## THE APPEARANCE OF THE OPTIC NERVE HEAD

Your doctor will use a variety of techniques to evaluate the health of the optic nerve to determine if there are any abnormalities of, or changes in, the appearance of the optic nerve head, including cupping, notching, or disc hemorrhages. Tried-and-true methods of examining the optic nerve head involve direct examination with the ophthalmoscope or the high-powered lens at the slit lamp. In each of these methods, the doctor is using a magnifying lens along with a powerful, well-focused light source to look through the pupil and study the details of the optic nerve head. In addition to directly examining the disc, the doctor may use some new, state-of-the-art techniques to determine whether the optic nerve is healthy

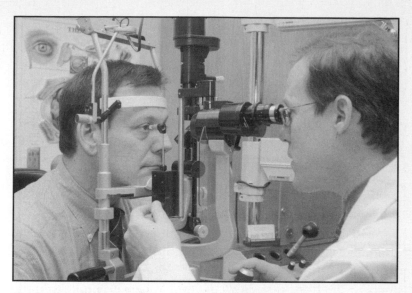

**Figure 22.** Measuring IOP using the Goldmann tonometer.

or whether there are signs of glaucoma damage. This is a significant advance in glaucoma management, since such technologies make it possible for the physician to know the precise location and extent of damage to the optic nerve as well as track changes in the optic nerve head over time. These new techniques will be described in chapter 13.

## MEASURING INTRAOCULAR PRESSURE (IOP)

By now, you are aware that elevated IOP is one of the major risk factors for glaucoma. Normal IOP ranges from 10 to 21 mm Hg.

### Goldmann Tonometry

Currently, the most accepted way to measure IOP is with Goldmann tonometry (figure 22). The Goldmann tonometer is an instrument attached to the slit lamp. Most slit lamps have tonometers.

Having your pressure measured with this test is quick, easy, and painless. The doctor will place a numbing eyedrop in your eye. The anesthetic may be premixed with sodium fluorescein, or the fluorescein may be applied with a paper strip. The fluorescein collects on the corneal surface, where it can be reflected by blue or fluorescent light. (A cobalt-blue light is used in Goldmann tonometry.)

To have your IOP checked with the Goldmann tonometer, you will position your chin on the slit lamp in front of the doctor and look straight ahead. You will see that the tip of the tonometer is illuminated with a cobalt-blue light. The doctor will slowly advance the tonometer toward you until it gently touches the front surface of the eye. When it is touching the cornea, the doctor will see two semicircles through the slit lamp. The doctor will then turn a dial on the tonometer until the two semicircles are touching or aligned in a particular way. When these semicircles are correctly aligned, this indicates that the IOP has been properly measured. The actual IOP measurement is taken from the dial that the physician has turned to align the two semicircles (figure 23).

Although Goldmann tonometry is the current standard, a number of factors could cause the IOP to be measured inaccurately. These include excessive or insufficient fluorescein, poor alignment of the semicircles, a thick or thin cornea, abnormal corneal curvature, and significant astigmatism.

### Diurnal (Daytime) and Nocturnal (Nighttime) IOP

IOP is not a static phenomenon; it varies throughout the entire twenty-four-hour period. Diurnal (throughout the day) and nocturnal (throughout the night) variations in IOP usually range from 3 to 6 mm Hg. Patients with IOP fluctuations

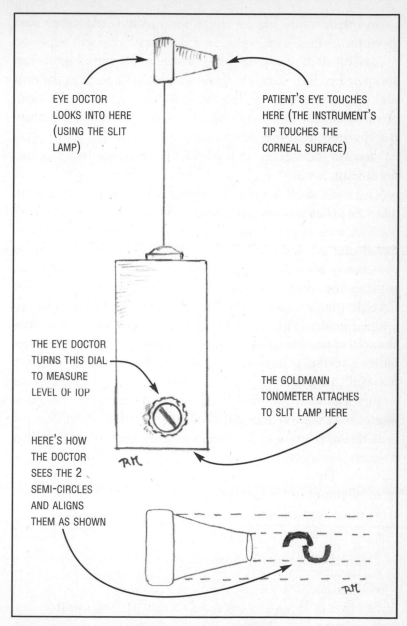

**Figure 23.** How the Goldmann tonometer works.

greater than 6 mm Hg are more likely to have glaucoma progression. In fact, some glaucoma patients have been reported to have IOP fluctuations of more than 30 mm Hg! When compared to individuals without glaucoma, glaucoma patients often have more variability in their diurnal IOP measurements, frequent differences between the two eyes, and diurnal IOP patterns that vary from one day to the next.

Diurnal and nocturnal IOP fluctuations may be more important than was thought in the past. We now know that for most people, IOP tends to be highest in the morning, within a few hours of waking. Still, several studies show that the IOP peak may be in the afternoon for some patients. It is now believed that diurnal and nocturnal fluctuations in IOP among glaucoma patients may be large and may be responsible, in part, for the damage related to glaucoma. Many doctors believe that large diurnal IOP fluctuation should be considered an independent risk factor for glaucoma progression. Furthermore, if a patient has a nocturnal lowering of blood pressure with an IOP that stays high overnight, this could be especially harmful to the eye.

In addition to the body's natural rhythms, IOP fluctuates throughout the day and night for other reasons. The following are some of the reported associations that tend to raise IOP (at least temporarily):

- Straining to lift something.
- Blinking hard and squeezing your eyes shut.
- Caffeine.
- Herbal tea.
- Tobacco.
- Steroids.
- Tight clothing around the neck, such as neckties.
- Lying down from the sitting position.
- Being in a head-down position.

- Looking up, if you have Graves' thyroid eye disease.
- Certain hormones: ACTH, glucocorticoids, growth hormone.
- Hypothyroidism.

Conversely, here are some factors that tend to lower IOP (at least temporarily):

- Aerobic exercise.
- A fat-free diet.
- Alcohol.
- Inflammation inside the eye (uveitis, iritis).
- Retinal detachment.
- Pregnancy.
- Certain hormones: progesterone and estrogen.
- Hyperthyroidism.
- Cold air.
- General anesthesia (most).
- Marijuana.
- LSD.

## Diurnal Variability of Glaucoma Medications

You will learn much more about specific glaucoma medications in the next chapter. But while we are discussing diurnal variations in IOP, it is important to note that there is variability in the efficacy of IOP-lowering drugs over a twenty-four-hour period. Each glaucoma medication has a time when it works at greatest effectiveness (peak) and least effectiveness (trough). The trough is usually just before the next dose of the medicine is taken.

### Diurnal Evaluations

When a patient's glaucoma appears to be worsening even though the IOP seems to be under reasonable control, a diurnal evaluation should be made. The doctor wants to determine the range of IOP and the amount of fluctuation, and avoid missing an IOP spike that could be overlooked with single readings. A nocturnal evaluation should be considered as well; however, this is difficult to carry out. Ideally, the doctor would use a device that would record a patient's IOP frequently throughout several twenty-four-hour periods, much as a Holter monitor assesses cardiac function. Unfortunately, such a device is not yet available. (Happily, this type of device is being developed; a prototype was presented to eye doctors in May 2003. See chapter 13 for more details.) However, it is still important for your doctor to measure the levels of IOP at different times of the day to document the range of pressures that exist. For example, you may be tested in the early morning, once in the afternoon, and then again in the evening. In some cases, your doctor may want to get a test called a diurnal curve. This test involves measuring the IOP every one to two hours throughout the day to determine the range of IOP levels.

No one knows the exact cause of the fluctuation in IOP. In most people, IOP is highest in the early-morning hours within a few hours of waking.

Doctors are becoming more convinced of the importance of measuring diurnal (daytime) and nocturnal (nighttime) IOP fluctuations. In a recent study, a group of glaucoma patients underwent twenty-four-hour IOP monitoring. In the majority of studied patients, doctors discovered IOP variations and IOP spikes that had not been found during office visits. As a result, the majority of these patients had their glaucoma management altered by their doctors. Clearly, the detection of significant variability in the IOP can help guide a doctor's decisions regarding treatment.

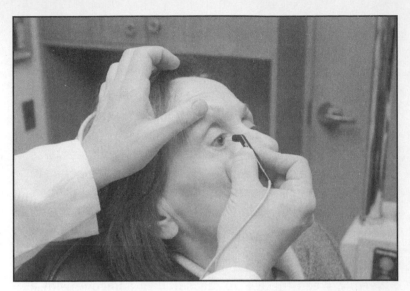

**Figure 24.** Measuring central corneal thickness (CCT): After a drop of anesthetic is applied to the eye, the ultrasound probe is gently touched to the central corneal surface. In less than a second, the ultrasound measures the CCT. In the most commonly used ultrasound for measuring CCT, the doctor sees a digital display of the CCT value in microns.

## THIN CENTRAL CORNEAL THICKNESS—AN IMPORTANT NEW RISK FACTOR FOR GLAUCOMA!

The measurement of central corneal thickness (CCT) and its importance in the management of glaucoma is a new and exciting phenomenon. The measurement of CCT is changing the way doctors evaluate IOP. In some—but not all—cases of glaucoma management, central corneal thickness is a crucial variable (figure 24).

Goldmann tonometry has been shown to be inaccurate when the corneal thickness deviates from the average of

540 to 550 microns. The National Institutes of Health (NIH) recently completed the Ocular Hypertension Treatment Study (OHTS). The purpose of this study was to determine whether early treatment could prevent or delay damage from glaucoma and to learn more about risk factors for glaucoma. I will be discussing this study in detail in chapter 12. But for now, a key finding was that thin (or thinner-than-average) central corneal thickness was shown to be a significant risk factor in the development of glaucoma among the studied patients with ocular hypertension (OHT). In addition, when a Goldmann tonometer is used to measure IOP in an eye with a thin cornea (low CCT), the pressure is underestimated. Thus, the patient and physician may have a false sense of security. Conversely, when the IOP is measured in someone with a thick cornea (high CCT), the IOP is overestimated.

No specific formula has yet been created that calculates the precise real IOP when the CCT deviates from average. A popular nomogram often considered by doctors for calculating the real IOP is the Ehlers nomogram:

• Ehlers nomogram: For every 100-micron deviation from the average CCT, add or subtract 7 mm Hg.

Though CCT is an accepted part of evaluating risk in patients with OHT, its use in patients with established primary open-angle glaucoma (POAG) is still being debated. A 2004 study of patients with established glaucoma by Herndon and colleagues published in the *Archives of Ophthalmology* shows that thinner CCT is associated with greater glaucoma damage. Ultimately—and hopefully soon—CCT will become a standard part of evaluating glaucoma patients as well as OHT patients.

## Noncontact Tonometer

The noncontact tonometer uses a puff of air to measure the pressure in the eye. This is commonly used in optometrists' offices and screening situations (since nothing touches the eye, and no numbing eyedrops are needed). The instrument shoots a puff of air into the patient's eye. The amount of time it takes for the air to flatten the cornea is measured. The elapsed time correlates directly with the IOP. The advantage to this test is that there is no contact with the instrument, no topical anesthetic is required, and the risk of corneal abrasion or infection is significantly reduced or eliminated. The disadvantage of noncontact tonometry is that the accuracy of the IOP measurement relative to Goldmann tonometry and other forms of contact tonometry is reduced.

While this may not be the most accurate screening device, it is a very valuable screening test that can indicate which people may have glaucoma or be more likely to develop glaucoma.

## Schiotz Tonometer

The Schiotz tonometer (figure 25) is a portable, easy-to-use instrument. Though less accurate than the Goldmannn tonometer, it allows doctors to measure IOP while a patient is lying down, faceup. This method of measuring IOP is usually reserved for patients who must be examined in bed or while lying down, as in the OR.

To measure IOP using the Schiotz tonometer, the doctor applies a drop of anesthetic to numb the eye, holds the instrument over the eye, and positions it onto the front surface of the cornea. The small plunger at the base of the tonometer slightly indents the cornea. The force that the tonometer requires to indent the cornea is directly proportional to the IOP. A thin, wand-like arm moves along a scale at the tonometer's upper

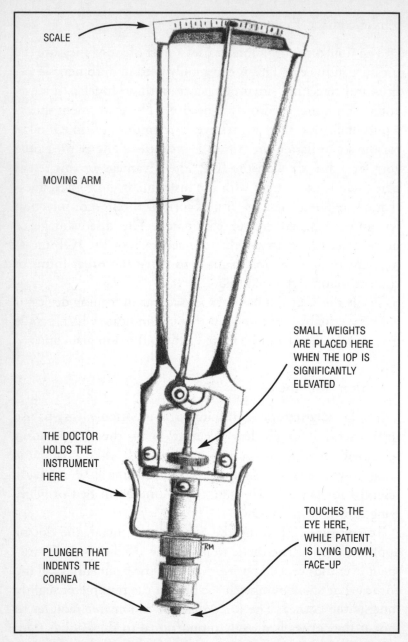

SCALE

MOVING ARM

SMALL WEIGHTS
ARE PLACED HERE
WHEN THE IOP IS
SIGNIFICANTLY
ELEVATED

THE DOCTOR
HOLDS THE
INSTRUMENT
HERE

TOUCHES THE
EYE HERE,
WHILE PATIENT
IS LYING DOWN,
FACE-UP

PLUNGER THAT
INDENTS THE
CORNEA

**Figure 25.** The Schiotz tonometer.

tip. The IOP is determined by reading the number off the scale (indicated by the wand-like arm) and using a conversion chart that accompanies the tonometer. Note that small additional weights can be placed on the tonometer if the IOP is significantly elevated and more force is required to indent the cornea.

### Pneumotonometer (Pneumatic Tonometer)

The pneumotonometer is a pencil-shaped instrument with a small disc-shaped sensor at its tip. The other end connects to tubing with pressurized air or gas. After the eye is given a numbing drop, the sensor touches the cornea. The force needed to push in or flatten the cornea is measured. This required force is used to calculate the IOP. The pneumotonometer is accurate and is often the preferred method to measure IOP when a patient has an irregular cornea.

### Tono-Pen

The Tono-Pen is a small, pencil-shaped device that is handheld, battery-operated, and very portable. In this technique, a numbing eyedrop is given. As the Tono-Pen touches the cornea, the cornea is indented. An electronic strain gauge creates an electrical signal that is used in the calculation of IOP. The Tono-Pen is often used in glaucoma screenings when a patient has an irregular cornea and when a patient cannot be examined at the slit lamp.

### Proview Eye Pressure Monitor (Bausch & Lomb)

The Proview tonometer was introduced in 2001. It was the first device created for at-home, self-monitoring of IOP and is easy to use. No eyedrop is required to numb the eye. You press the small tubelike device onto your partially closed eyelids, not onto the eye itself. The reliability and accuracy of this device will vary among users. Instruction by a physician is strongly advised. In addition, this device should be used under the direction and supervision of a doctor who is able to interpret the IOP readings and assess their reliability and accuracy.

## VISUAL FIELD TESTING

Determining and monitoring the visual field are crucial aspects of the detection and management of glaucoma. By monitoring the patient's visual field, doctors are monitoring whether or not vision is being lost. You might think that a patient could easily detect a loss of sight without having to be tested, but that is *not* the case. In glaucoma, it is the peripheral (side) vision that is most commonly affected first. Loss of peripheral vision can go unnoticed at the early stages. In fact, loss of peripheral vision can often go undetected until significant glaucoma damage is present! This inability of a person to notice peripheral vision loss is one of the reasons that glaucoma often goes undetected. In addition, patients often assume that because they can see well straight ahead, their eyes must be healthy. This is a bad assumption. (One notable exception to the "rule" that peripheral vision is lost first in glaucoma may occur in normal-tension glaucoma, or NTG, in which the visual field in the central—rather than side—portion is more commonly affected in the early stages.)

Visual field testing has evolved tremendously over the years. Currently, the state-of-the-art visual field test is the Humphrey automated perimeter (figure 26). In this test, you sit in a darkened room in front of a concave screen and are given a buzzer to hold. Your head is positioned in front of this concave screen, or "bowl," that displays a sequence of lights in a variety of positions throughout the visual field. You are told to stare straight ahead. A computer program flashes lights of different intensi-

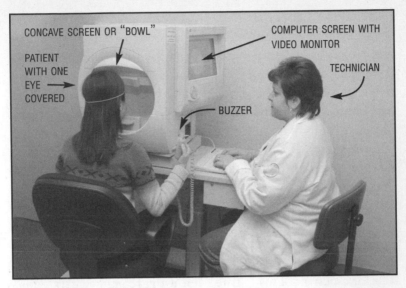

CONCAVE SCREEN OR "BOWL"

COMPUTER SCREEN WITH VIDEO MONITOR

PATIENT WITH ONE EYE → COVERED

TECHNICIAN

BUZZER

**Figure 26.** Visual field testing with the Humphrey automated perimeter, performed in a darkened room.

ties at different points on the screen. Whenever you detect a flash of light you press the buzzer. One eye is tested at a time, while the other eye is covered. The technician monitors your eye movements throughout the test by looking at a video monitor on the perimeter's computer screen. You are encouraged to blink (to keep the eye well-lubricated) and to concentrate while staring straight ahead. Since the test requires concentration, it is best to do the visual field in a quiet environment with few distractions. At the completion of the test, the visual field results are printed for you and your doctor to review.

The visual field program also determines if your test results are reliable or not. That is, the machine can tell if you are looking around and searching for the dots, instead of staring straight ahead and using your peripheral vision. Looking around (termed fixation losses) makes the test unreliable. A false positive occurs when you press the button as if you have seen a dot of light when there was none. (This may indicate a "trigger-happy" patient.) A false negative occurs if you have not pressed a button when shown a flash of light that should have been easily detected. This pattern may indicate inattentiveness or a shift in head position. In analyzing the visual field test, the doctor must look not only at the results but also at these reliability parameters: fixation losses, false positives, and false negatives. If the results are unreliable, the test should be repeated another day. Before repeating the visual field test, the doctor should explain why the previous test was unreliable and provide additional instructions.

*One visual field test is usually not enough to reliably and definitively make a diagnosis or even establish an adequate baseline.* Often it takes three visual field tests to establish a reliable baseline for a patient. This is true even if the reliability parameters are good. This is because visual field testing results vary for a number of reasons. Visual field tests may be inaccurate if you are tired or distracted, if you're not seated comfortably in front of the machine, if an incorrect eyeglass prescription is used to choose the lens through which you look during the test, if the technician setting up the visual field did not properly position you or failed to dim the lights, or if he or she neglected to tell you to stare ahead at the fixation light.

The main point to remember is that *you should not panic if you have one abnormal visual field test.* It does not necessarily mean that your optic nerve is abnormal or that there has been a progression of your glaucoma. A repeat visual field test will usually be scheduled.

Visual field testing has advanced greatly in recent years. New visual field tests allow earlier detection of glaucoma. I will be describing these in chapter 13.

To properly diagnose and monitor glaucoma, three vital factors must be examined and monitored diligently: the level of

IOP; the appearance and health of the optic nerve head; and peripheral vision (the visual field). Chapter 5 has covered the basic ways in which these factors are monitored. Fortunately, recent advances in technology now allow doctors to monitor these factors in much more sophisticated ways. All these advances and the newest technologies that are most likely to be found in the office of a glaucoma specialist are discussed at length in chapter 13.

# Chapter 6

# Medication

Once glaucoma (or ocular hypertension that warrants treatment) has been diagnosed, the doctor will begin treatments—usually with topical medications (eyedrops). Over the past decade, a number of new medications have become available to treat glaucoma. Because of these advances, the treatment of glaucoma has changed dramatically.

Before the introduction of the newest glaucoma medications, patients commonly began therapy with a topical beta-blocker if there were no reasons the medication should not be prescribed. Beta-blockers decrease the rate at which aqueous is produced by the eye. At that time, Timoptic (generic name: timolol) was often the first drug to be prescribed by the doctor. If the intraocular pressure (IOP) was not sufficiently lowered using Timoptic, an additional medication—usually Propine 0.1 percent, twice per day—would be added. If those medications failed, a third and possibly a fourth medication would be given. Among those medications was pilocarpine, which is used *four times per day*!

Treatment with so many medications was not an ideal solution for the patient *or* the doctor. Knowing *what* to take and *when* to take it could become very confusing for the patient. And the more medications, the greater the chance of side effects. With four different eyedrops, it was often unclear as to which medication was causing a bad side effect. And compliance with all those drops was an impossibility!

Today physicians can choose from new types of glaucoma medicines that are far more effective than the older medications, much better tolerated, and, depending on the type of medication, may be used only once per day! This means that compliance will improve dramatically. Even if a patient ultimately requires more than one type of eyedrop, the treatment regimen is likely to be far simpler now than before the newer products became available.

## HOW LOW SHOULD YOU GO?

In addition to deciding which medication to prescribe, the doctor must also decide what the target IOP should be. He or she may have in mind either a specific IOP level or range, or a percentage of IOP reduction to aim for. It is important to keep in mind that there is no specific number that has been found to be *the* level at which a person's eye is safe from glaucoma-related damage. Some people require an IOP between 8 and 10 mm Hg, while others can tolerate IOPs above 21. The eye doctor must be the one to choose *each patient's unique IOP target*, since what is a safe IOP level for one patient may not be safe for another. Among many variables, the doctor strongly considers the following factors when determining the target IOP range: amount of glaucoma damage (cupping); IOP levels at which damage occurred; rate at which the glaucoma is worsening; patient's age, race, lifespan, and family history.

Once the target IOP range or goal has been set, the doctor will begin medical therapy. He or she will try to achieve the target IOP with the simplest therapeutic regimen possible. The simplest regimen to comply with is *monotherapy*—treatment with just one drug. So ideally, the doctor will strive to find a single drug that can achieve the desired results.

The stability of your glaucoma is monitored in large part by checking the appearance of the optic nerve head and measuring the visual field. If these appear to be deteriorating, your doctor will accordingly modify and lower the target IOP.

*Remember that the goal of treatment is to preserve your sight and quality of life by preventing optic nerve damage. If there has already been damage to the optic nerve, it cannot be reversed.*

## GLAUCOMA MEDICATIONS

There are at least five classes of drugs and many combinations of medications that can be used to control IOP. Despite the availability of such a large selection, most doctors will prefer monotherapy, starting you on one drug and having you remain on that medication alone for approximately one month. The doctor will want to determine if that *one* medication, on its own, can bring your IOP to the target range that has been chosen for you individually. If the IOP target is not reached with the single medication, instead of adding another drug the doctor will probably change to a different medication and reassess. As I mentioned earlier, it is easier for a patient to faithfully and consistently take one medication rather than multiple medications. Having to take only one medication facilitates patient compliance, and *patient compliance is key*! Monotherapy also tends to be less expensive, and reduces the likelihood of side effects. However, if monotherapy is unable to control the IOP adequately, a second medication will be considered. In addition to medications, other alternatives include argon laser trabeculoplasty (ALT), selective laser trabeculoplasty (SLT), and glaucoma filtration surgery (trabeculectomy). The choice depends on your unique profile: amount of nerve damage, visual field, age, IOP, IOP target or goal, central corneal thickness (CCT), life expectancy, medical health, tolerance of glaucoma medications, degree of compliance with medications, and other factors.

## What Are These Medications and How Do They Work?

Medications to lower IOP work in two basic ways: They either reduce the amount of fluid produced by the eye or increase the amount of drainage out of the eye. Of course, the ways in which each medication achieves these effects differ. Some medications lower IOP by achieving *both* effects (dual mechanism of action).

Medications that increase the drainage of aqueous from the eye include:

- Hypotensive lipids, a category that can be broken down further into prostaglandin analogs (such as Xalatan, Travatan, and Rescula), and prostamide compounds (such as Lumigan).
- Alpha-2 agonists (such as Alphagan P and brimonidine).
- Cholinergic agents (such as pilocarpine).
- Sympathomimetics (such as Propine).

Medications that decrease the rate at which aqueous is produced within the eye include:

- Beta-blockers (such as Timoptic, timolol, Betoptic S, Betagan, and Ocupress).

- Alpha-2 agonists (such as Iopidine, Alphagan P, and brimonidine).
- Carbonic anhydrase inhibitors (such as Trusopt, Azopt, Neptazane, and Diamox).

Medications come in a variety of forms: eyedrops, pills, liquids, gels, and intravenous solutions. However, the most common form of glaucoma medication is the eyedrop.

I will use the remainder of this chapter to describe each of the major categories of glaucoma drugs and the most commonly prescribed products. You can find a complete listing of all the glaucoma drugs available at the time this book is being published in appendix C.

## HOW TO PLACE AN EYEDROP IN YOUR EYE

Proper placement of your eyedrops onto the eye will ensure that you obtain the maximal effect with the fewest side effects.

After an eyedrop is placed on the eyeball, the medication drains from the surface of the eye into tiny drains in the corner of the eye (near the nose): the puncta. Blinking your eyelids causes more medication to flow from the surface of the eye into the puncta. Placing a finger over the puncta for one or more minutes will ensure that each eyedrop is properly absorbed by the eye and *minimally* absorbed by the rest of the body. This is nasolacrimal occlusion (NLO).

Here are the steps to follow:

1. Wash your hands.
2. Tilt your head slightly back and look up toward the ceiling.

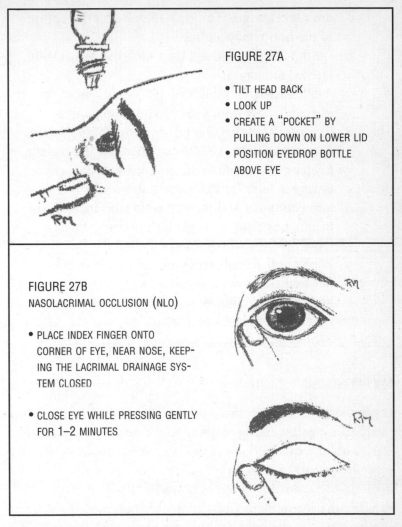

**Figure 27.** Giving yourself an eyedrop and nasolacrimal occlusion (NLO) technique.

3. Use your index finger to gently pull down your lower lid, forming a sort of pocket.
4. Position the bottle of eyedrops over this pocket.
5. Gently squeeze the bottle so that only one eye-

drop is released. (For Xalatan, tapping the bottom of the bottle may suffice.)

6. Do not let the bottle's tip touch the eye, eyelid, lashes, or fingers.
7. Avoid excessive blinking; this causes more medication to flow from your eye into the puncta.
8. Place your index finger on the corner of the eyelids closest to your nose. This will occlude the puncta, keeping the medication on your eye and not allowing it to enter the puncta (from which it goes into your nose and throat). Hold your index finger in this position, with gentle pressure, for one or more minutes with your eye closed.
9. Wipe or rinse any excess medication from the eyelids and skin.
10. Wait 5 to 15 minutes or more before placing any other eyedrop onto your eye.

## HYPOTENSIVE LIPIDS

Instead of starting our discussion with the oldest glaucoma medications and working our way to the newest, I am going to start with the medications many glaucoma doctors prescribe most frequently. For glaucoma, the most prescribed *type* of medication worldwide is the hypotensive lipid.

With the introduction of the new hypotensive lipid glaucoma drugs in the mid-1990s, the therapeutic choices for glaucoma were vastly improved. The doctor's search for one medication that will effectively and safely help you reach your target IOP became much easier.

The beta-blockers (Timoptic, timolol, Betoptic S, Betagan, Ocupress, and so forth), which had been standard first-line therapy before the introduction of the hypotensive lipids, have the potential for major side effects, including reduced blood pressure, fatigue, shortness of breath, worsening of heart failure, depression, impotence, hair loss, and the masking of low blood sugar symptoms in diabetic patients. This side effect profile makes the beta-blockers less than ideal for many patients.

The hypotensive lipids have far fewer side effects than the beta-blockers, and most are taken only once a day, making them more convenient than most of the beta-blockers as well. A doctor will often—but not always—select a hypotensive lipid as a way to initiate glaucoma treatment.

In my own practice, if the hypotensive lipid I have chosen as my first choice for therapy (monotherapy) is unable to adequately control the IOP, I often switch to one of the other hypotensive lipids before choosing a drug from another category. Recent studies have confirmed that if a patient is not responding well to one hypotensive lipid, that same patient may respond adequately to a different hypotensive lipid. *To optimize compliance, monotherapy is a goal worth striving for!*

There are three major hypotensive lipids: Xalatan, Lumigan, and Travatan. A fourth hypotensive lipid is Rescula. Rescula, however, is much less effective than the other major three lipids and is used twice per day, not once. For these reasons, Rescula is generally not considered to be one of the three major, potent hypotensive lipids. Instead, it is more often used as adjunctive therapy or a less desirable choice within the hypotensive lipid family.

The three major hypotensive lipids are divided into two types: prostaglandin analogs and prostamide compounds. Xalatan and Travatan are prostaglandin analogs. Lumigan is a prostamide compound.

I will begin by describing Xalatan, the first prostaglandin analog to become available. Xalatan came on the market in the mid-1990s.

## Xalatan (latanoprost)

Xalatan is currently the gold standard in glaucoma therapy. It is approved by the Food and Drug Administration (FDA) as monotherapy for glaucoma, the hypotensive lipid that has been in use for the longest period of time, and the drug that the FDA would compare any new drug to (the definition of *gold standard*). Since its introduction in 1996, it has become and remains the most prescribed glaucoma medication in the United States and internationally.

Xalatan is a pro-drug. This means that the medication exists in an inactive form while in the bottle. As it enters the eye, the inactive form of the medication is converted to an active form, or metabolite. The drug binds to a receptor in the eye called the FP receptor.

Xalatan lowers IOP by increasing uveoscleral outflow. This is an alternate route by which aqueous fluid leaves the eye—a route that does not involve the movement of aqueous through the trabecular meshwork. Xalatan has been shown to reduce IOP by 27 to 34 percent. Moreover, it provides good twenty-four-hour IOP control. Unlike Timoptic, Xalatan is able to maintain a steadily reduced pressure over months and years without IOP drifting upward.

Side effects include hyperemia (redness of the eye) in 5 to 15 percent of patients. The iris may change color due to an increased production of melanin, and you may experience increased growth of your eyelashes. (Eyelashes often become longer and thicker.) The eyelids and the skin below the eyes may darken. There have also been some reports of inflammation in the eye with Xalatan. A doctor may need to avoid using this medication if you have a history of iritis or other intraocular inflammation such as cystoid macular edema (CME), or have a history of a complicated cataract removal with a posterior capsule that is not intact. Overall, and for most patients, however, Xalatan is safe, effective, and well tolerated.

At present, Xalatan is the *only* hypotensive lipid that is FDA-approved as first-line therapy for glaucoma. It is interesting to note that most glaucoma specialists have been treating glaucoma with Xalatan as first-line therapy for years. It is comforting to glaucoma specialists, other ophthalmologists, and optometrists that the FDA has now confirmed the safety and efficacy of Xalatan as a first-line therapy. In addition, because Xalatan has been proven safe and effective for a significant number of years, many doctors are convinced of this medication's long-term safety for their patients. The other hypotensive lipids have not been available for this length of time, and their long-term safety and efficacy have not been substantiated in the way that Xalatan's have.

Apart from its high efficacy rate and its low incidence of side effects, what makes Xalatan a breakthrough drug is the fact that it achieves such significant IOP lowering while only being taken *once a day*. Studies have shown that using Xalatan more than once per day results in less IOP lowering than with a once-daily dosing. The reasons for this are not known.

Patients usually take Xalatan in the evening, before bed. I usually advise patients to invert the bottle when it is placed above the eye and then tap the bottle without squeezing. This routine generally releases just one drop of medication. For patients with difficulty administering drops, the makers of Xalatan (Pfizer) recently created a small device called Xal-Ease, which assists you in dispensing just one drop directly onto the eye. In addition, I tell patients to close the eyelid immediately after applying the medication and keep it closed for at least one minute to make sure it is well absorbed. To further ensure absorption and reduce the amount of drop that goes down the nose and throat, nasolacrimal occlusion (NLO) is recommended. This technique involves placing gentle pressure on the inner corner of the eye by the tear duct (see figure 27).

Xalatan is currently available in one size, which is a 2.5 cc bottle. Each bottle contains a six-week supply. Unlike other drugs in this category, Xalatan currently requires refrigeration while it is unopened. Once the bottle has been opened, it remains stable at room temperature for six weeks. If you receive samples of Xalatan from your doctor, you will notice that they have a twelve-month expiration date rather than the eighteen-month expiration date that is on the regular bottle. That is because doctors' samples have been approved for storage at room temperature, while bottles at the pharmacy must be stored in the refrigerator. Efforts are under way by Pfizer to have the FDA remove the requirement that Xalatan be refrigerated. For convenience, Xalatan is now available in a multipack with three individual bottles in one package.

Outside the United States, Xalatan is also available in a combination medication form called Xalcom. (In some countries, this drug is named Xalacom.) Xalcom and Xalacom contain Xalatan plus timolol 0.5 percent. Amazingly, worldwide sales of Xalatan/Xalcom have now reached a billion dollars annually. This is the first ophthalmic medication to achieve this level—ever!

### Rescula (unoprostone)

The next hypotensive lipid to be released was Rescula, another prostaglandin analog. This is a much less potent hypotensive lipid and its ability to lower IOP is significantly less than the other hypotensive lipids. Initial studies showed that Rescula reduced IOP 14 percent compared to 28 percent with Xalatan. In my practice, I have found that the IOP-lowering effect of Rescula is similar to that of Trusopt. It is generally used as an additive medication, in combination with other medications. When used as monotherapy, it is often in patients who are intolerant of or nonresponsive to the other glaucoma medications. Rescula does have a role in the treatment of glaucoma, but that role is a limited one.

Rescula, which lowers IOP by increasing uveoscleral outflow, is taken twice a day. It requires no refrigeration and is well tolerated by most patients. It does have the usual side effects seen with other hypotensive lipids (eyelash growth, iris pigmentation, and so on), but these side effects tend to be less than is seen with other hypotensive lipids.

### Travatan (travoprost)

Travatan was released March 16, 2001. Like Xalatan, it is a pro-drug. Travatan has a higher affinity (tendency to bind) to the FP receptor than any other prostaglandin analog. It reduces IOP by increasing uveoscleral outflow, and it is taken only once a day. It requires no refrigeration.

In a twelve-month study comparing Travatan and Xalatan, subjects had their IOPs measured at 8:00 A.M., 10:00 A.M., and 4:00 P.M. There was no statistically significant difference between the two drugs at 8:00 A.M. or 10:00 A.M. However, at 4:00 P.M., Travatan was more effective in lowering IOP than Xalatan. Like other hypotensive lipids, Travatan is more effective than Timoptic. Furthermore, initial studies of this drug showed (erroneously) that Travatan appeared to be more effective in lowering IOP in African American patients. To date, this has not been substantiated by other research and is believed *not* to be an accurate conclusion. Studies are now ongoing to determine whether these findings can be duplicated. Travatan is safe, effective, and well tolerated, with IOP-lowering effects and side effects similar to Xalatan's.

In the near future, Alcon will be releasing a *new*, once-daily combination medication that is made of Travatan plus timolol

0.5 percent. This new drug, which is awaiting FDA approval, has been named Extravan.

### Lumigan (bimatoprost)

Lumigan was also approved by the FDA and released on March 16, 2001. It is unlike the other hypotensive lipids in that it is a prostamide compound. Most research shows that Lumigan acts on a different receptor than the other hypotensive lipids. Also unlike other hypotensive lipids, Lumigan has a *dual mechanism of action*. It increases uveoscleral outflow and also increases outflow by the trabecular meshwork. Lumigan is a once-a-day medication, and it requires no refrigeration. It is not a pro-drug, which means that the drug itself is the active agent (compared to Xalatan and Travatan, which convert to an active agent in the eye). Research presented in March 2004 at the American Glaucoma Society's annual meeting has shown that Lumigan may actually be a pro-drug. Further research is being conducted to resolve this controversy.

In studies comparing Lumigan and Timoptic, Lumigan was able to reduce IOP by approximately 33 percent versus 23 percent for Timoptic. In a study comparing Lumigan's diurnal daytime IOP control against Xalatan's, there was less fluctuation throughout the day with Lumigan. Additionally, Lumigan appears to be equally effective in African Americans and other ethnic groups.

Like the other hypotensive lipids, Lumigan has very few systemic side effects. The side effects it does have include those that are common to all hypotensive lipids: eyelash growth, hyperemia (redness), and iris color change. Compared to the other hypotensive lipids, Lumigan does cause a significantly higher incidence of redness in the eye (hyperemia). But in virtually all patients who use these medications, the hyperemia was described as mild or trace and was usually tolerated.

\*     \*     \*

Recent studies have attempted to compare these hypotensive lipid glaucoma medications and their ability to lower IOP. A study by Dr. Robert Noecker and co-workers reported in the January 2003 issue of *American Journal of Ophthalmology* compared Xalatan and Lumigan in a six-month, randomized clinical trial. The study was a well-designed, multicenter, investigator-masked, parallel-group study. This study found that both medications were safe and effective, but concluded that Lumigan was able to lower IOP more than Xalatan in a statistically significant way, with Lumigan lowering mean IOP more than Xalatan by approximately 1.5 mm Hg (range of 0.9 to 2.2 mm Hg). Noecker's data showed that Lumigan lowered IOP more than Xalatan at every time point throughout the study. Data from this study showed that Lumigan was able to achieve lower target IOPs more often that Xalatan—especially when IOP targets were below 15 mm Hg. Further analysis of the data from this study showed that Xalatan's nonresponse rate (the rate at which patients responded poorly or not at all to a medication) was two to three times greater than Lumigan's. Though Lumigan was shown to produce more ocular hyperemia (redness) than Xalatan, the discontinuation rate (number of patients needing to stop the medication because of an adverse reaction) was the same for both medications: 4.5 to 5.0 percent.

A 2003 study by Dr. Richard Parrish and co-workers reported in the May 2003 issue of *American Journal of Ophthalmology* compared Xalatan, Lumigan, and Travatan in a twelve-week, randomized, parallel-group, evaluator-masked study. Dr. Parrish's study concluded that the IOP-lowering effect of the three hypotensive lipids was essentially the same. No statistically significant difference in IOP-lowering effect was found. The study found that the drugs' IOP-lowering effects were not statistically different. The study was not designed to say that the three medications are equivalent; proving equivalence is a more difficult task. The study did note that significantly fewer patients reported ocular hyperemia (redness) with Xalatan. However, the reported hyperemia was mild, in the lower ends of the redness scale for all three of the medications—including Lumigan.

Clearly, more research is needed to clarify the advantage of one hypotensive lipid over the other.

## BETA-BLOCKERS

Prior to the introduction of the hypotensive lipids, initial therapy in treating glaucoma was dominated by the beta-blockers. Beta-blockers decrease the rate at which aqueous is made within the eye. There are two general categories of beta-blockers: *selective* (specific to one receptor) and *nonselective.*

Beta-blockers have been and remain popular because they are effective and have been tested over time. Their pressure-lowering effect is often quite predictable, and they are often well tolerated.

The major beta-blockers include:

- Timoptic (timolol)—nonselective, BID (twice a day).
- Timoptic XE—nonselective, QD (once a day).
- Betoptic S (betaxolol)—selective, BID.
- Ocupress (carteolol)—nonselective, BID.
- OptiPranolol (metipranolol)—nonselective, BID.
- Betagan (levobunolol)—nonselective, BID.

Because of the potential for adverse side effects with beta-blockers, patients with asthma, chronic obstructive pulmonary disease (COPD), and some other forms of cardiovascular and pulmonary disease should avoid beta-blockers in the treatment of glaucoma. Patients who are already taking an oral beta-blocker such as Inderal may not experience the full IOP-lowering effect of the topical beta-blockers. In other words, these patients may get less of an IOP-lowering effect than those who are not on oral beta-blockers.

Another important and often overlooked concern that doctors must consider with any beta-blocker eyedrop is the potential for nocturnal hypotension (nighttime fall in blood pressure). This may adversely affect the optic nerve's circulation at night and allow glaucoma progression.

### Timoptic (timolol)

For the twenty years prior to the release of Xalatan, Timoptic was considered the gold standard in the treatment of glaucoma. Available in either a twice-a-day solution or a gel-type solution (Timoptic XE) taken once a day, Timoptic has proven long-term efficacy (approximately 24 to 34 percent reduction of peak IOP) and a good safety record. Most people tolerate the medication well. However, there are many potential side effects related to Timoptic, as with all the beta-blockers. These side effects include shortness of breath, hypotension (low blood pressure), headache, fatigue, depression, reduced libido, impotence, insomnia, and other cardiac and pulmonary side effects.

Timoptic XE is timolol in a gel form that is used once daily. As the solution contacts the tears, a gel is formed. As a gel, the medication has enhanced contact time with the cornea. There are fewer systemic side effects with Timoptic XE as compared to Timoptic BID (twice daily) solution, since the body has less exposure to the beta-blocker. Its effectiveness is about the same as Timoptic BID; however, patient compliance with this XE form of Timoptic is probably better because it only needs to be taken once a day. A brief blurring of vision is more often reported by patients using the gelform rather than the solution.

### Betoptic S (betaxalol)

Betoptic S is the most widely prescribed selective beta-blocker. It is selective in that it affects only beta-1 (cardiac) receptors—and not beta-2 (pulmonary) receptors—resulting in fewer pulmonary side effects. Overall, Betoptic S is a very well-tolerated beta-blocker, but is less effective than Timoptic in reducing IOP.

## ADRENERGIC AGONISTS

Adrenergic agonists are a class of glaucoma medications that vary greatly in their ability to lower IOP. Within this class, there are two main categories: *nonselective* adrenergic agonists (including epinephrine and Propine) and *selective* alpha-2 adrenergic agonists (including Iopidine, Alphagan, Alphagan P, and brimonidine).

Nonselective agents, such as epinephrine and Propine, though popular for decades, are no longer widely used because of significant side effects that include eye irritation, redness, conjunctivitis (pinkeye), blurred vision related to pupil dilation or macular edema (swelling in the central area of the retina), angle-closure glaucoma, increased heart rate, and hypertension.

The selective adrenergic agonists grew rapidly in popularity because of their effective lowering of IOP and minimal side effects. Today *Alphagan is the second most prescribed glaucoma medication in the world.* (In the United States, Alphagan has been replaced by Alphagan P; brand-name Alphagan is no longer available. Recently, a generic version of Alphagan—brimonidine—was introduced. *There is no generic version of Alphagan P.*)

The first drug in this family of selective alpha adrenergic agonists was clonidine, introduced in 1983. Clonidine lowers IOP by reducing aqueous humor production. Unfortunately, clonidine was found to have serious side effects such as hypotension (low blood pressure), lowered pulse, and sedation. As a result, clonidine was deemed unsuitable for the routine treatment of glaucoma.

The second drug, Iopidine (apraclonidine), was developed and found to reduce IOP significantly without the life-threatening side effects of clonidine. Unfortunately, Iopidine has significant ocular and systemic side effects such as allergy, eyelid retraction, pupil dilation, dry mouth, headache, and fatigue that limit its usefulness. Today, Iopidine is used primarily to blunt or avoid the IOP spikes that can follow routine laser trabeculoplasty, laser iridotomy, and laser posterior capsulotomy. One drop is given one hour before and immediately following the laser treatment to help avoid these post-laser IOP spikes.

### Alphagan and Alphagan P

With the introduction of Alphagan (brimonidine), a safe, well-tolerated, and effective drug within this family of medications became available.

Alphagan is a highly selective alpha-2 adrenergic agonist with good IOP-lowering ability—without the significant side effects of its predecessors. Alphagan has a *dual mechanism of action*: It reduces aqueous production and increases uveoscleral outflow. Its maximum effect takes place over two hours, and it is taken BID (twice a day) or TID (three times a day).

Alphagan has a similar efficacy as Timoptic at peak (when the effect of the medicine is at its highest) but is less effective than Timoptic at trough (just before the next drop is due to be used, when the medicine's effect is least). Alphagan has minimal cardiac and pulmonary side effects—fewer than the beta-blockers. Alphagan is not contraindicated in patients with cardiopulmonary disease. It is generally avoided in children because of the risk of hypotension and apnea (short periods when breathing stops). Because of its effective and safe profile, Alphagan is popular worldwide.

As noted, in the United States, Alphagan has now been replaced with Alphagan P. This new form of Alphagan was introduced by Allergan in August 2001. Alphagan P has the same effectiveness as Alphagan, but the delivery vehicle has been changed to include a safer and better-tolerated preservative: Purite. Purite is a gentle preservative that is often found in artificial tears. In addition to better tolerability, Purite improves the absorption of the active ingredient in Alphagan P. This effect is termed enhanced bioavailability and allows the concentration of the active ingredient, brimonidine, to be lowered. A lower concentration of medication (0.15 percent versus 0.2 percent) is delivered in each dose. Despite this lowered concentration, the IOP-lowering effect is the same. However, due to the reduced concentration, Alphagan P produces fewer bodily side effects than Alphagan (and generic brimonidine). This has made the medication safer overall.

Side effects of Alphagan P include ocular allergy, burning sensation, stinging, blurred vision, lid retraction, dryness of the mouth, hypertension, and visual disturbance. Overall, however, this is a very well-tolerated medication.

Many doctors consider Alphagan or Alphagan P to be an excellent second choice for IOP control after the hypotensive lipids. Though Alphagan P is often added to a hypotensive lipid, it can be used alone as well.

Finally, it is interesting to note that several studies of brimonidine usage in animals showed a neuroprotective effect (protecting the optic nerve from damage, independent of its IOP-lowering effect on the eye). To date, neuroprotection with brimonidine in humans is not proven.

## CARBONIC ANHYDRASE INHIBITORS

This category of drugs reduces the amount of aqueous fluid made within the eye by inhibiting carbonic anhydrase, an enzyme necessary for the production of aqueous humor by the ciliary body. Carbonic anhydrase inhibitors (CAIs) have been available for many years in oral form. Specifically, these include Diamox (acetazolamide) and Neptazane (methazolamide). These oral medications are effective at lowering IOP, but are poorly tolerated over time and can lead to significant electrolyte imbalances. The CAIs can create a lowering of potassium and the development of kidney stones. In addition, there have been reports of aplastic anemia associated with the oral form of carbonic anhydrase inhibitors. These medications are typically contraindicated in patients with renal (kidney) disease and must be used with caution in patients on certain cardiac and hypertension medications. Other systemic side effects include fatigue, loss of appetite, weight loss, nausea, depression, loss of libido, tingling sensations, and a metallic taste when drinking carbonated beverages.

The topical forms of CAIs (Trusopt, Azopt) do not show these significant side effects. Overall, topical CAIs are less effective in lowering IOP than Timoptic, but more effective than Betoptic. Studies have shown IOP reductions of 17 to 23 percent at peak. Topical CAIs are often used as adjunctive therapy, which means that they are taken in conjunction with other medications.

### Trusopt (dorzolamide)

Trusopt (dorzolamide) is a topical carbonic anhydrase inhibitor. It lowers IOP by reducing aqueous production. Its usual IOP-lowering effect is 3 to 5 mm Hg. Trusopt is used two or three times a day.

With Trusopt, there are no acid–base or electrolyte disturbances reported as there are with the oral CAIs such as Diamox and Neptazane. Trusopt has minimal or no effect on blood pressure or heart rate and is not associated with aplastic anemia. There have been only rare reports of kidney stones related to Trusopt. Other side effects were reported in less than 2 percent of patients. These included headache, ocular stinging, and some reports of fatigue. There are no pulmonary or cardiac contraindications to this medication.

### Azopt (brinzolamide)

Azopt is the other major topical carbonic anhydrase inhibitor. It is a suspension and is therefore thicker than Trusopt. For this reason, Azopt—as compared to Trusopt—is more often associated with a temporary blurring of vision. Like Trusopt, Azopt reduces aqueous production to lower IOP. Usually, a reduction in IOP of 4 to 5 mm Hg can be seen. However, because Azopt is pH-balanced, there is less stinging than with Trusupt. Azopt is taken two or three times a day.

## COMBINATION MEDICATIONS

Since it is not uncommon to prescribe more than one medication to control IOP, pharmaceutical companies often market products that have two medications already combined. A distinct advantage of a combination medication over a regimen of several different medications is improved compliance. One such product is Cosopt, which is a combination of Trusopt (dorzolamide) and Timoptic (timolol). Its mechanism of action is to decrease aqueous humor production to lower IOP.

Cosopt is taken twice a day. It is easier to use than two separate medications, since it requires taking only one medication twice a day rather than one medication twice a day and the other three times a day. However, it is important to remember that because this drug contains both medications, the side effects are equal to those of each medication combined. The contraindications related to each apply to this drug.

A recently released drug is Xalcom, a combination of Xalatan and timolol. (In some countries, this drug is named Xalacom.) At present, Xalcom is not available in the United States, but it is widely distributed elsewhere in the world. Xalcom is made by Pfizer (formerly Pharmacia).

New combination medications are currently being developed. These include Lumigan plus a beta-blocker (currently unnamed), Alphagan plus a beta-blocker (Combigan), and Travatan plus timolol (Extravan).

## GENERIC DRUGS: ARE THEY REALLY JUST AS EFFECTIVE?

Generic glaucoma medications continue to grow in popularity. Generics offer potential cost savings to patients and insurers covering drug costs. These cost savings are important because they could allow some patients to have their glaucoma managed with medicines despite an inability to afford the brand-name drugs.

Doctors and patients need to be cautious in their use of generics, however. Most important, there is a lack of data to confirm therapeutic and safety equivalence. Without this information, it is uncertain that a patient will do as well with the generic as with the brand name. The FDA requires that the generic drug mimic the branded medication in its concentration of active ingredient, dosage, and route of administration. Unfortunately, the FDA allows the preservatives and buffering agents to vary from the branded medication. These seemingly small differences may have a great impact on the tolerability and effectiveness of the generic medication and allow generic equivalents to vary greatly among themselves. Also, there are many generic manufacturers. You may receive your medication from a different manufacturer each time a prescription for the generic is filled. This leads to problems in assuring and maximizing patient stability.

Proponents of generics believe that the cost savings outweigh all the concerns. They argue that generics allow patients to pay less for their medicines and/or for their drug plan co-pay. In addition, there is less cost for medication to the health care system overall.

But it is important to keep in mind that drug cost is only one factor. There are also hidden costs to consider. With less money spent for brand-name drugs, less money becomes available for the development of new medicines (research and development) by the brand-name manufacturers. (Generic drug makers have little or no interest in developing new medicines.) Also, doctors will often need to see their patients who switch to generics several extra times to confirm that the generic is working as well as the brand-name product. In fact, the patient on generic medications may need a number of extra patient visits with the doctor to deal with issues of tolerability and efficacy.

Overall, generics offer *potential* cost saving benefits that are appealing in many ways to patients, insurers, and the health care system in general. But the risks associated with using generics cannot be overlooked. Clearly, these risks would be minimized if generic drugs were required to demonstrate therapeutic equivalence to brand-name medicines. However, at this time, the makers of generic drugs are not required to provide data confirming therapeutic and safety equivalence. Therein lies the problem. *Remember: Generics are not necessarily equivalent.*

At the time this book is being written, the newest generic glaucoma medication being introduced is brimonidine, the active ingredient in Alphagan and Alphagan P. This generic medication is being produced by Bausch & Lomb. At present, there is no generic equivalent for Alphagan P, which is the brimonidine-Purite formulation.

## COMPLIANCE

Once a treatment regimen has been created, compliance is vital. *Compliance* is the term used to describe patients' ability to properly follow a doctor's directions for the treatment of their condition—in this case, glaucoma. *Noncompliance* describes the inability to properly follow the treatment plan prescribed by the doctor. Because most glaucomas are chronic (ever-present) conditions, usually have no symptoms, and the loss of sight usually comes on slowly, people with glaucoma are often noncompliant with their medications. But noncompliance is extremely dangerous to the health of your eyes and can cause you to lose your sight. It is critical that you work with your glaucoma doctor to create a treatment plan that you will be able to follow as prescribed.

If you are diagnosed with glaucoma, keep the following facts in mind:

- Your doctor has said you have glaucoma.
- You have read this book.
- You understand what glaucoma is.
- You understand that glaucoma can cause you to lose sight *permanently*, even if you are unaware that it is happening.

Therefore, you know that using your treatment as prescribed is your best chance of holding on to your sight.

## BECOMING AN ACTIVE PARTICIPANT IN YOUR GLAUCOMA TREATMENT

- Ask questions. Make sure you understand why you need to take the medication and what the medication is doing for you.
- Learn about the possible side effects of your medication. Report any side effects or allergic reactions to your doctor promptly. Between visits, keep notes about things you need to discuss with your doctor.
- Understand that an allergic reaction to a medication may be related to the preservatives it uses. Discuss this possibility with your doctor when reporting allergic reactions. You and your doctor can consider an alternative medication with no preservative or less preservative.
- Know the proper way to take your eyedrops. Learn about the spacing of medications and nasolacrimal occlusion techniques (described earlier in this chapter) to minimize bodily side effects.
- Talk to your doctor. Be sure your doctor listens to you *and* that you are listening to your doctor.
- Take notes during your visit.
- When you visit your doctor, bring along a relative or friend. Often, it is easier to remember and understand what your doctor has explained and instructed if you have someone else to help listen and ask questions. Later, they can help you recall things you may have forgotten. In the resources section of this book, you will find recommendations for reliable organizations that can provide the kinds of information you may need to supplement what you hear from your doctor.

- Discuss your lifestyle with your doctor: your time of waking, eating, sleeping, and so forth. This information will help your doctor create a treatment schedule that works for you.

- Ask your doctor (or your doctor's assistants) for a written list of your medications and the times to use them. Write down your medication routine. Include the drug name, time to use, frequency, and dosage. Make a chart. Keep a log.

- Try to use your medications at the same time each day. Link the use of your medication with something else you do routinely at a certain time of day or night. For example, a drop that is used before bed can be used each night just before you brush your teeth.

- Maintain a good working relationship with your doctor. Consider yourselves a team. Work with your doctor to find a routine of medicines that you can comply with. Together, you can tailor a treatment plan that suits your unique needs and schedule. But this will take effort on both your parts. There needs to be two-way communication.

- *Do not be afraid to ask questions.* Ask your doctor as many questions as you need to. Be sure you understand what you need to do, why you need to do it, and how to do it properly.

# Chapter 7

# Laser Surgery

A *laser* (an acronym for "light amplification by stimulated emission of radiation") is a highly concentrated and powerful beam of light. Lasers are used in many ways in today's world. Lasers can cut metal and glass with extreme precision. They are used in virtually every U.S. retail store to scan bar codes during checkout. They are used in CD players to play music. Lasers can reshape the cornea to correct vision (LASIK surgery).

Laser surgery is often used to treat glaucoma. For some glaucoma patients, laser surgery may be one of the first treatment steps recommended by their doctor. Other patients may be guided toward laser treatment if medication does not reduce the intraocular pressure (IOP) to a sufficient degree, or if medications fail to maintain an adequately controlled IOP over time. (Remember that some glaucoma medications can gradually lose their effectiveness over time. Timoptic, in particular, is known for this phenomenon, called drift.)

There are a number of different types of lasers. The three

main types used in the treatment of glaucoma are the argon, YAG, and diode. These lasers are named by the elements within them that help generate the beam of light.

Doctors use laser light in a variety of ways to treat glaucoma. In some cases, laser light is applied to the eye's drainage system (trabecular meshwork) to improve the flow of aqueous through the drain. The most commonly performed laser procedure of this type has been argon laser trabeculoplasty (ALT). The newest version of laser trabeculoplasty, however, is the selective laser trabeculoplasty (SLT). SLT uses the YAG laser instead of the argon laser. *SLT is rapidly gaining acceptance as doctors become more experienced with its use and are finding results comparable to ALT.* SLT will be described in chapter 15 since it is a recent innovation in laser surgery.

In another laser procedure, the doctor makes a small opening in the iris to allow aqueous to reach the drain. This procedure is performed in patients with a narrow or closed drainage angle—specifically, those who have narrow angles (and are predisposed to angle-closure glaucoma) or who have angle-closure glaucoma. This procedure, called laser peripheral iridotomy (LPI), is most commonly performed with a YAG laser but can alternatively be performed with an argon laser.

If your doctor recommends that you undergo laser surgery, the exact type will depend on the particular type of glaucoma you have. In fact, the specific type of laser and the exact way in which the laser procedure is performed will be unique to *you*.

## ARGON LASER TRABECULOPLASTY (ALT)

The use of lasers to treat the drainage angle of a glaucoma patient was first considered a realistic option in the 1970s. Initial laser treatments were designed to make small punctures or openings in the drainage system (trabecular meshwork). This proved unsuccessful in achieving and maintaining a lowered IOP.

The popularity of laser trabeculoplasty in the treatment of elevated IOP grew throughout the 1980s. Finally, in 1990, the Glaucoma Laser Trial published its results. This study confirmed ALT to be a successful and effective first-line therapy for glaucoma.

Since the concept of ALT was first introduced in the 1970s, many different laser types—using many different wavelengths of laser light—have been used to treat the drainage angles of patients with elevated IOP. In addition to the argon laser, the krypton, Nd:YAG (neodymium: YAG), diode, and, most recently, frequency doubled Nd:YAG laser (for selective laser trabeculoplasty) have been used.

### How Does ALT Work?

It was initially believed that during ALT, small punctures were being made in the drainage system (trabecular meshwork). We now know that this is not the case. Laser energy being applied to the drain does not penetrate its full thickness; no puncture is made. Instead, the laser energy creates a small *thermal burn* on a very superficial portion of the drainage system. In this way, ALT can actually increase the ease (facility) of outflow by 50 percent. There are two main theories as to why this is so.

The first theory is that these laser scars create a small amount of shrinkage where they are applied. Therefore, there is a stretching, or tension, placed on the beams within the trabecular meshwork that lie *between these small scars*. The stretching of the tissue between each of the small superficial laser scars causes the spaces within the meshwork to open more widely. Aqueous is able to pass through more easily, and IOP is reduced.

The second theory is that the argon laser creates a biochemical change in the trabecular meshwork that reduces the resistance to outflow. For example, the laser could actually cause the cells within the trabecular meshwork to divide and healthy new trabecular cells to be made. These new cells could then migrate into the treatment areas and repopulate these zones with healthy, normal trabecular meshwork.

Although the exact mechanism by which ALT works is not fully understood, it is clear that the laser energy creates a change in the cells and tissues of the trabecular meshwork (in addition to many superficial, small, thermal scars within the meshwork). Over the course of three to six weeks, these changes—whatever they are—can cause the aqucous to flow more easily from the eye. As a result, IOP is lowered.

## Success Rates with ALT

In studies looking at all forms of glaucoma being treated with ALT, initial success rates range from 60 to 97 percent. Within that range, it has been found that patients who have *not* undergone cataract surgery, patients who have open-angle glaucoma, and/or patients who have pseudoexfoliation (exfoliative glaucoma) respond better to ALT than people who have other forms of glaucoma.

In the short term (approximately one year), studies have reported an 80 to 97 percent success rate for ALT in the treatment of *primary open-angle glaucoma*, or POAG (usually closer to 80 percent). Though ALT is likely to lower the IOP and help bring glaucoma under control, success with ALT does not necessarily mean that medications can be completely eliminated. In fact, only 58 percent of patients are able to reduce their medications after ALT, and only 5 percent are able to eliminate medications altogether.

Unfortunately, the IOP-lowering effect of ALT diminishes over time. After one year, the success rate associated with ALT is about 80 percent. With each additional year, however, the failure rate increases by 7 to 10 percent. Studies reveal that after five years, the probability of success is approximately 57 percent. Other studies are less optimistic and estimate a five-year success rate of only 35 percent. Generally, the overall success rate for ALT after five years is 35 to 44 percent. Does this mean that the effects of ALT can never last beyond five years? Not at all. In 32 percent of patients, ALT is successful after ten years.

An important study related to the success of ALT is the Advanced Glaucoma Intervention Study (AGIS), also described in chapter 12. This study was designed to look at the effectiveness of ALT compared to trabeculectomy in patients with advanced and worsening glaucoma despite maximal medical therapy. African American patients undergoing ALT were found to have slightly better preservation of visual function (as determined by visual acuity and visual field testing) as compared to African American patients undergoing trabeculectomy. Caucasian patients did slightly better with trabeculectomy as compared to ALT. Over time, the difference between the outcomes of the ALT and trabeculectomy groups diminished. However, the study does suggest that African American patients could possibly do better with ALT than trabeculectomy.

In *exfoliative glaucoma*, the success rate with ALT is initially very high at 97 percent, with an average IOP lowering of 12 to 17 mm Hg. However, the effects of ALT often do not last. At one year, the success rate is 50 to 70 percent. Uncommonly, IOP after ALT in these patients can be higher than baseline. (Remember that in people with exfoliative glaucoma, IOP often responds poorly to medications but has a very high initial success rate with ALT.)

In *pigmentary glaucoma*, ALT success is reported to be from 44 to 80 percent at one year. By the sixth year, the success rate is 45 percent. An important finding here is that unlike patients with POAG, patients with pigmentary glaucoma, who tend to be younger, respond better to ALT than their older counterparts.

In *aphakic* (the eye's natural lens is removed, with no intraocular lens implant or IOL) and *pseudophakic* (the eye's natural lens is replaced with an IOL) patients, the success rate of ALT is reduced. The overall success rate is approximately 60 to 85 percent, but with an average of only 6 mm Hg reduction in IOP. It is unclear why ALT is less successful in patients who have undergone cataract surgery. However, it is generally known that ALT is more effective in an individual glaucoma patient if ALT is performed *before* cataract surgery.

It is possible to perform ALT in patients who have undergone a previous trabeculectomy. The initial success rate in these patients is approximately 70 percent.

Patients who are *not* good candidates for ALT (those in whom it will be partially effective or ineffective) are those with significant peripheral anterior synechiae (PAS), or scarring of the angle; a recessed angle (perhaps related to trauma); or ICE syndrome (iridocorneal endothelial syndrome—see chapter 4). In addition, ALT is generally ineffective in patients with uveitis. In fact, uveitis patients may experience a significant elevation in IOP related to a reactivation of uveitis. In patients with chronic angle closure, many glaucoma specialists believe that at least half the angle must be open to treat this condition successfully with ALT without creating a permanent elevation in IOP. Patients with angle recession respond poorly to ALT over the long run.

### Can ALT Be Repeated?

For most doctors performing ALT, one session of ALT consists of thirty-five to fifty laser spots distributed equally over half (180 degrees) of the eye's drainage system. (Remember that the eye's drain is situated in the angle, where the cornea and iris meet. The drain is, therefore, circular. Like all circles, it has 360 degrees; half of a circle is 180 degrees.) A second ALT session is needed if the IOP is insufficiently lowered. A second session would consist of thirty-five to fifty spots over the untreated half of the eye's drain (180 degrees).

After ALT has been performed over 360 degrees of the angle (the entire circumference of the eye's drainage system), retreatment is often ineffective. The initial success of ALT after 360-degree treatment is estimated to be approximately 33 percent, and often this success is short-lived. Of greatest significance is that approximately 17 percent of patients undergoing ALT after the eye's entire 360 degrees of drain have been previously treated end up with a *significant rise* in IOP.

### Can ALT Be Used as a Primary Therapy?

The answer is yes. The Glaucoma Laser Trial looked at the efficacy of initial treatment for POAG with ALT versus medical therapy with beta-blockers such as Timoptic. Studies showed that 44 percent of patients were controlled with ALT alone after two years, and that patients who had undergone ALT (often, but not always) needed fewer glaucoma medications.

### What Are the Effects of Race, Sex, and Age on ALT?

African American patients appear to have a greater success rate based on visual field and visual acuity in the long term as compared to Caucasian patients. For patients under the age of forty, there is a significant failure rate with ALT. In 60 percent of these patients, ALT can produce uncontrolled IOP elevation and perhaps lead to the requirement of filtration surgery within two years. Similarly, congenital and juvenile-onset glaucoma show low success rates with ALT.

## ALT: The Procedure

The first step for your doctor is to obtain informed consent from you, the patient. In my practice, I usually then administer a drop of Alphagan P or Iopidine to blunt any possible post-laser spikes in IOP. Anesthetic eyedrops are applied to the treatment eye (and sometimes to the untreated eye to prevent inadvertent blinking), and you are seated in front of the laser with chin on the chin rest and forehead firmly against the forehead rest.

To perform this procedure, the physician uses a three-mirrored lens, which sits comfortably on the eye. The lens is lubricated with methylcellulose, a thick, viscous material that is used as a coupling solution. It is this material that actually touches the eye and makes rotation of the lens possible without being uncomfortable, while minimizing the risk of corneal abrasion. The placement of the lens is completely painless.

The doctor positions the mirrored lens on the eye in such a way as to be able to visualize the drainage angle to be treated (figure 28). Usually, the doctor will treat 180 degrees (half the eye's circular drainage system) during the first session of ALT. The choice of which 180 degrees—which half of the circular drain—varies among doctors.

During the treatment, thirty-five to fifty spots are applied and distributed evenly over 180 degrees. Typical laser settings are as follows: fifty-micron spot size, 0.1-second duration, and a power of approximately 0.6 watt. The exact power settings for the laser vary for each individual and with the amount of pigmentation present in the angle. The endpoint for the laser treatment is your doctor seeing a blanching or a small bubble formation on the surface of the drain (trabecular meshwork).

ALT is painless and takes approximately two to five minutes. Most patients describe feeling a sense of impact for each of the spots given, but they do not describe the sensation as

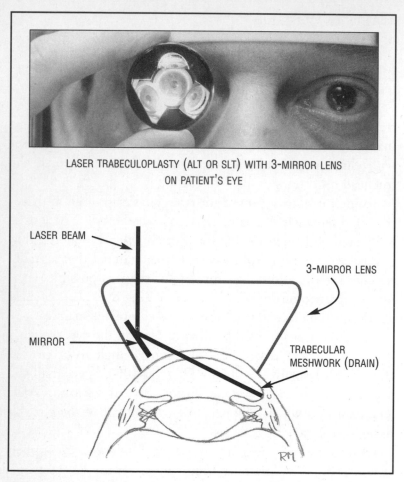

LASER TRABECULOPLASTY (ALT OR SLT) WITH 3-MIRROR LENS
ON PATIENT'S EYE

LASER BEAM

3-MIRROR LENS

MIRROR

TRABECULAR
MESHWORK (DRAIN)

RM

**Figure 28**. Laser trabeculoplasty (ALT or SLT): Using a mirrored lens, the doctor views the angle under high magnification with the slit lamp. The laser beam is focused very precisely onto the trabecular meshwork.

being painful. In other words, patients are aware that a laser treatment is being done but are completely comfortable.

Following the ALT, your doctor will probably rinse the excess methylcellulose out of your eye to reduce the blurring and ask you to sit and wait for thirty to sixty minutes. At the end of that time, the IOP is checked. If there has not been a significant IOP rise, you will be discharged with instructions to use a topical steroid drop (such as prednisolone acetate 1 percent, Lotemax, or Alrex) or a nonsteroidal drop (like Acular) four times a day for four to seven days. Follow-up varies among individual patients, but a typical pattern for exams is one hour, one day, one week, and four to six weeks. The effects of ALT cannot be fully judged until four to six weeks have passed.

### The Postoperative Period

Immediately after ALT, you may experience blurred vision. This is related to the methylcellulose that was used as a coupling agent, and will disappear as the substance is eliminated from the eye. Light sensitivity, irritation, redness, and inflammation may also be present. There are no restrictions on your activities. No eye patch is required.

During the initial four-to-six-week period, when the doctor is waiting to see if the ALT worked, you will probably continue to use some or all of your pre-laser glaucoma medications. The exact medication regimen will depend on many variables, including the post-laser IOP level. During this post-laser period, most patients must continue on glaucoma medications because the laser treatment may not become effective for four to six weeks. Discontinuing IOP-lowering medications before this time could prove dangerous!

### Who Should Undergo ALT?

Among glaucoma specialists in the United States, it is generally accepted that for most forms of open-angle glaucoma, ALT (or the newer form of laser trabeculoplasty—selective laser trabeculoplasty, SLT, which will be described in chapter 15) should be considered before proceeding with traditional filtration surgery. Clearly, the choice to do ALT is based upon a complete evaluation that includes an assessment of the patient's risk factors: type of glaucoma, age, race, ability to tolerate medications, and previous laser and surgical history.

Patients who should *not* undergo ALT (in whom it is contraindicated) are those who have a closure of the angle by peripheral anterior synechiae scar tissue.

### Complications of ALT

The incidence and severity of complications will vary based upon the individual patient and type of glaucoma. One potential complication is a long-term worsening of the glaucoma. Overall, 3 percent of patients with POAG can get worse following ALT. Second and more common is an acute rise in IOP. However, IOP increases after ALT are usually blunted and/or prevented by your doctor pretreating with Alphagan P or Iopidine. Another possible complication is uveitis or iritis (inflammation inside the front chamber of the eye). After ALT, uveitis is usually mild and short-lived and is treated with topical steroids (or nonsteroidals) for four to seven days. In some cases, however, the inflammation can be severe, leading to the formation of PAS (scar tissue inside the angle).

An uncommon (immediate) complication is the development of corneal burns, in which the laser energy has been defocused and inadvertently applied to the cornea. These burns usually heal within a few days and can generally be avoided when the doctor has good visualization of the angle to be treated.

Another possible complication is bleeding. Since the argon laser is a heating laser, this is a rare event. However, should a small amount of bleeding occur, the physician need only press firmly against the eye with the mirrored lens; the bleeding should stop.

Finally, progressive visual field and vision loss should be considered among the complications associated with ALT. It is possible—although very uncommon—that a significant IOP rise will follow ALT treatment. If this occurs, a patient with a significantly compromised or fragile optic nerve could experience visual field and central vision loss.

### Trabeculoplasty with Other Lasers

Most commonly, laser trabeculoplasty is performed using argon blue or green laser light. However, as I mentioned in the beginning of the chapter, other lasers can also perform this procedure, including the krypton (red), continuous wave (neodymium: YAG), diode, and frequency doubling (FD) Nd:YAG. Most exciting of these is the FD Nd:YAG, better known as selective laser trabeculoplasty. This will be discussed in greater detail in chapter 15.

## LASER IRIDOTOMY (LASER PERIPHERAL IRIDOTOMY, OR LPI)

Laser iridotomy is a procedure in which laser energy is used to make an opening through the iris, allowing aqueous to move easily from the posterior chamber into the anterior. This tiny passageway allows aqueous to bypass its normal route—from its origin at the ciliary body, beneath the iris, and through the pupil into the anterior chamber. Instead, the aqueous travels directly from the ciliary body through the iris opening (iridotomy) into the anterior chamber—then out the drain. LPI is the preferred method for managing numerous angle-closure glaucomas that have some degree of pupillary block.

As mentioned previously, some physicians call this procedure a peripheral iridectomy because a small portion of the iris is being removed, while others call it a peripheral iridotomy because a small opening, or hole, is created within the iris. Throughout this book, I use the term *iridotomy* for this laser procedure because I believe it to be more accurate (although both terms are technically correct).

Before lasers were around, patients with angle-closure glaucoma, mixed-mechanism glaucoma, or severely narrow angles had to undergo surgical iridectomy (surgical removal of a small portion of iris) in the operating room. This surgical procedure is associated with numerous potential complications including a significant risk of hemorrhage, infection, wound leakage, and cataract. In addition, anesthesia was required to perform the procedure.

In the 1970s, when the argon laser became available commercially, surgical iridectomy was in large part replaced with laser iridotomy. With this technical advance, the procedure could be performed easily with a laser, avoiding surgical intervention in the operating room. With the advent of the Nd:YAG laser (YAG, for short), argon became a distant second choice. The YAG used much less energy, required fewer laser applications, and resulted in a lower rate of iridotomy closure (loss of patency).

The argon laser produces thermal energy that is delivered directly into the iris tissue itself. In great contrast, the YAG laser does not create a thermal burn or injury to the iris. Instead, it creates a photodisruption and related shock waves, which then mechanically rupture the tissue without heat. Argon laser iridotomy often results in areas of iris atrophy around the created hole, but this does not occur around iridotomies made with the YAG laser. In addition, because the YAG laser does not have a coagulative or thermal effect on the iris, bleeding is more common than with the argon. (For this reason, in a glaucoma patient who requires LPI but is receiving anticoagulants such as aspirin, Plavix, or Coumadin, and cannot discontinue them before the laser, an argon LPI could be preferred over a YAG LPI to reduce the risk of bleeding.)

Today the laser of choice for iridotomy is the YAG. Overall, the energy required to do the iridotomy is significantly reduced, and the ease of doing the procedure is significantly increased.

### Who Should Have Laser Iridotomy?

One common indication for laser iridotomy is an obstructed or occludable angle in a person who does not have glaucoma, but who is at risk for developing angle-closure glaucoma (narrow angles). Other indications include pupillary block with angle closure, pupillary block with narrow occludable angles, chronic angle closure, combined angle-closure glaucoma, incomplete surgical iridectomy with lack of patency (closing of the hole), suspected malignant glaucoma, pupillary block after cataract extraction, and nanophthalmos. Contraindications include corneal diseases, disorders that would not allow visualization of the iris, and an anterior chamber that is completely flat (there is a great chance of damaging the cornea should a laser iridotomy be performed).

### LPI: The Procedure

You must first provide informed consent. Your doctor will discuss potential complications with you. These include:

- The possibility of incomplete iridotomy.
- The possible need for a repeat session to complete the iridotomy.
- A rare, late closure of the iridotomy.
- Iris bleeding (primarily with YAG).
- Postoperative IOP elevation.

- The possibility of continued IOP elevation which requires medical and/or surgical treatment.
- Persistent, intermittent glare (described as an annoying awareness of light shining into the eye through the iridotomy).

Other possible complications include mild postoperative inflammation, light sensitivity, blurring, and redness. Blurred vision (immediately after the laser) is generally related to the pilocarpine drops that are typically given beforehand. Blurred vision is also often due to the methylcellulose coupling agent used during the procedure to keep the lens from irritating the surface of the eye. If you are on aspirin, Coumadin, or other medications that promote bleeding, the doctor will usually speak with your internist to see if these medications can be safely discontinued for one week prior to the laser.

After informed consent is obtained, you are given pilocarpine 1 or 2 percent drops every five minutes (usually a total of three drops) or until the pupil is constricted. This creates a thinning of the peripheral iris so that a thin portion of iris can be identified as the laser iridotomy site. Slight blurring of the vision may be noted as well as a "brow ache" or headache with the pilocarpine. Alphagan P or Iopidine (or a beta-blocker, if there is no contraindication) is given thirty minutes before laser therapy to blunt a potential postoperative IOP rise.

When you are seated at the laser, a drop of topical anesthetic is applied and the iridotomy lens is placed on the eye using a methylcellulose coupling agent. The lens of choice for peripheral iridotomy is the Abraham lens. The Abraham lens has a high-power "button" or zone that allows the physician to see the area of iris to be treated in great magnification. This increases the concentration of energy at the iris and decreases the amount of energy at the level of the cornea. With this high-power lens, the laser beam is very well focused. Posterior to the

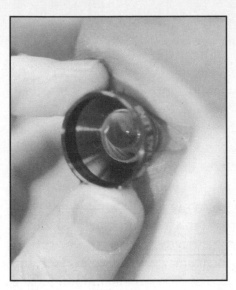

**Figure 29.** Laser peripheral iridotomy (LPI) using the Abraham lens: Using the Abraham lens, the peripheral iris is viewed under high magnification using the slit lamp. The laser beam is focused on the peripheral iris, generally in an area of the iris that is hidden beneath the upper lid. The laser's energy is applied to this area until a microscopic opening in the iris is achieved.

site of focus, the beam is more rapidly defocused, which reduces the chance that there will be injury to any structures behind the iris such as the lens capsule, the lens, or the retina.

The YAG laser usually completes the iridotomy in one to five shots, depending on the thickness of the iris, degree of pigmentation, and power settings used. (If an argon laser is used, many more applications will be required.) The procedure is completely painless, but you usually feel an "impact" with each laser shot. The location of the iridotomy is usually beneath the upper lid and slightly off-center, toward the temple. The position of the iridotomy is such that there is minimal chance of postoperative glare or double vision. Choosing a naturally thin area makes it easier for the laser to penetrate the iris. By avoiding iris blood vessels, the chance of bleeding during the procedure is reduced. If bleeding does occur, the doctor may press the lens firmly and briefly onto the eye to stop it. If this is not successful, the doctor may use the argon laser to cauterize the bleeding vessel.

## Argon Laser Iridotomy

Although the Nd:YAG laser is the laser of choice for this procedure, the argon laser may sometimes be required. This technique generally requires many more applications of laser to the iris, but it is an excellent option for patients who cannot discontinue anticoagulant therapy (such as aspirin or Coumadin) before the laser iridotomy. Unlike the YAG laser, the argon laser has a heating (or thermal) effect, which reduces the chance of bleeding during the procedure. However, for the person with a light blue iris, the argon is more difficult because the energy is poorly absorbed by a lightly pigmented iris. In these patients, the YAG laser is clearly the laser of choice.

Argon laser iridotomy patients may experience iris bleeding, localized cataract, immediate post-laser IOP elevations, inflammation, or closure of the iridotomy. Large postoperative IOP elevations are typically short-lived and occur in only 30 percent of patients. Pretreatment with Alphagan P or Iopidine greatly reduces the chances of such postoperative IOP elevations.

Closure of the iridotomy is a complication that mainly occurs with an argon laser iridotomy and can occur in 30 percent of cases. If the laser iridotomy is found to be open at the four- to six-week examination, it can be expected to remain open indefinitely. Uncommonly, closure of the iridotomy could occur in patients with extreme uveitis (inflammation) or neovascularization. Repeat laser iridotomy may be needed in such patients.

## Postoperative Management

Postoperative management is tailored to the individual. You usually receive topical corticosteroids for several days to a week after the procedure. The classic follow-up is: examination and IOP check at one hour, one day, and one week after treatment. At a subsequent visit, once the iridotomy is confirmed to be

patent (open), the eye is dilated to reduce the chance of peripheral anterior synechiae and to allow examination of the retina.

### What About Residual Glaucoma?

After a laser peripheral iridotomy is completed, your IOP
may still be elevated. In these cases, it is best to wait at least a
month (when possible) before deciding on further intervention such as whether laser trabeculoplasty or filtration surgery
would be required to control the IOP.

## OTHER LASER PROCEDURES

### Laser Goniopuncture

This procedure is often associated with nonpenetrating
glaucoma filtering surgery (described in chapter 15) when
there is a small portion of tissue separating the filter from the
anterior chamber. Following the nonpenetrating glaucoma filter surgery, aqueous will begin to filter through a very thin,
membranelike tissue. If the IOP is insufficiently lowered by
the nonpenetrating surgery, the YAG laser is used to make an
opening in this membrane to enhance flow of aqueous from
the anterior chamber. Following goniopuncture, the aqueous
no longer needs to filter through the thin layer of tissue. Instead, the aqueous passes directly out of the anterior chamber,
escaping more easily. There is less resistance to aqueous outflow and a lowered IOP.

### Laser Suture Lysis (LSL)

Laser suture lysis is a procedure to cut a suture that has been
placed onto the eye during filter surgery (trabeculectomy). It is
performed in post-trabeculectomy patients who need to have

their IOP lowered. The procedure is usually performed with the argon laser and a suture lysis lens, which is placed onto the anesthetized conjunctiva of the eye. A krypton laser may also be used and may be preferable if there is blood overlying the suture.

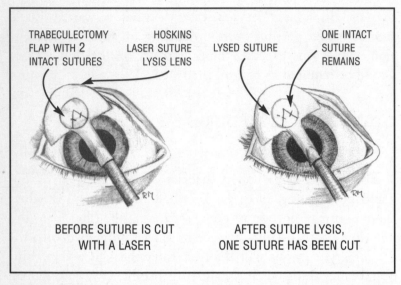

TRABECULECTOMY FLAP WITH 2 INTACT SUTURES

HOSKINS LASER SUTURE LYSIS LENS

LYSED SUTURE

ONE INTACT SUTURE REMAINS

BEFORE SUTURE IS CUT WITH A LASER

AFTER SUTURE LYSIS, ONE SUTURE HAS BEEN CUT

**Figure 30.** Laser suture lysis (LSL): This figure shows the Hoskins laser suture lysis lens being used to view the trabeculectomy flap and its sutures. Under the high magnification of this lens and the illumination of the slit lamp to which the laser is attached, laser energy is applied to the suture to be cut.

## Argon Laser Iridoplasty (ALI or Gonioplasty)

This laser procedure is done to alter the configuration of the peripheral iris, particularly in the far periphery of the iris—the iris that lies closest to the trabecular meshwork (drainage angle). ALI involves the placement of small areas of thermal energy onto the extreme peripheral iris, causing localized iris contraction. As the iris tissue contracts, the iris is pulled away from the drain and further opens the angle. This procedure is beneficial in patients who have anatomically narrow angles despite a patent peripheral iridotomy. Specifically, ALI is used in an uncommon condition called plateau iris syndrome (see chapter 4).

## Cycloablation

• *Cyclophotocoagulation (transscleral)*: One method of reducing IOP is to reduce the amount of aqueous that the eye makes. To do this, the ciliary body itself is treated because it is the ciliary body that makes the aqueous. This procedure is typically reserved for patients who have failed other, more traditional treatments such as medications, laser trabeculoplasty, and filtering surgery (trabeculectomy). In this procedure, the diode laser is used to apply thermal energy through the sclera to deliver its energy into the ciliary body. The diode laser for this procedure is of two basic types: contact and noncontact. In the *contact* diode, a probe is used to deliver the laser energy to the surface of the eye. In the *noncontact* form, the laser energy is delivered without touching the eye. In each case, the goals are the same: to damage the ciliary body and reduce its ability to produce aqueous. The reduced production of aqueous causes IOP to fall.

• *Endophotocoagulation* is similar to cyclophotocoagulation in that both techniques involve laser treatments on the ciliary body to reduce aqueous production. With cyclophotocoagulation, the energy is applied transsclerally; with endophotocoagulation, the instrument is placed directly inside the eye (through a surgical incision) so that the energy is applied directly to the ciliary body.

Endophotocoagulation can be performed under direct visualization. This procedure is called endoscopic cyclophotocoagulation (ECP). ECP can be accomplished using the Endo Optiks endoscopic cyclophotocoagulation laser released by Medtronic Ophthalmics in 2002. The device is the size of a small twenty-gauge needle. It is inserted through an incision in the cornea or at the limbus (the junction of the sclera and cornea, overlying the trabeculor meshwork). ECP can be performed during phacoemulsification (ultrasound cataract surgery) or in a separate procedure. (Advocates of this procedure believe that direct visualization of the ciliary body is important when treating the ciliary body. The ciliary body is not directly visualized in transscleral cycloablation.)

In the ECP treatment, laser energy is directly applied to the ciliary body tissue (called ciliary processes) between 180 degrees (half of the entire ciliary body tissue) and 360 degrees (full circumference). Studies have shown that treatment of 180 degrees decreases IOP by 25 percent. Treatment of 275 degrees decreases IOP by 35 percent. Further study of the ECP procedure is needed.

*Chapter 8*

# Traditional Surgery

When intraocular pressure (IOP) cannot be adequately controlled using medications or laser, filtering surgery (trabeculectomy) is usually the next step. Trabeculectomy is a type of filtration surgery during which the doctor opens the conjunctiva to reveal the sclera (the hard, white shell of the eye) beneath. Within the sclera, the doctor creates a small, hinged "flap." This allows a new drainage channel to be created from the inside to the outside of the eye. As aqueous fluid percolates out through this new drain, it creates a bleb—a small cystlike elevation on the surface of the eye. The bleb is actually the reservoir of aqueous on the surface of the eye. From this bleb, aqueous is reabsorbed into the bloodstream.

During the first half of the twentieth century, surgeries to reduce IOP in glaucoma involved cutting through the full thickness of the sclera. These procedures, known as full-thickness filtration surgeries, often resulted in many complications, such as hypotony (IOP that is too low), flat anterior chamber, cataract, a thin, leaky bleb, and endophthalmitis (a very serious eye infection).

Trabeculectomy, a partial-thickness (*not* full-thickness) filtration surgery, is used in both open-angle and closed-angle glaucomas. Its goal is to reduce IOP, thereby preserving vision. It is important to understand that trabeculectomy *cannot* reverse glaucoma-related damage or improve vision. However, it *can* help preserve the vision that remains. The surgery may also make it possible to eliminate or reduce glaucoma medications. (Some patients do have improved vision after surgery—when their glaucoma eyedrops, which were blurring vision, are stopped.) Uncomplicated, first-time trabeculectomy has a high success rate (75 to 90 percent) and often allows a patient to significantly reduce or eliminate glaucoma medications. Trabeculectomy is usually done on one eye at a time, not bilaterally.

## TRABECULECTOMY

Once a decision has been made to do a trabeculectomy, the first step is to discuss the risks and benefits with your doctor and provide an informed consent for the procedure. In addition, you must receive medical clearance from your internist. Anticoagulation medications such as aspirin, oral nonsteroidal anti-inflammatory medications, Coumadin, and certain glaucoma medications (including pilocarpine and carbachol) should be discontinued prior to surgery.

Trabeculectomy takes approximately twenty to forty-five minutes and is done in the operating room. It might take longer if you have had previous surgery and scar tissue is present. The procedure is usually performed under local (not general) anesthesia. You receive intravenous sedation for relaxation and injections of local anesthetic around the eye. Sometimes only topical anesthesia (numbing drops and gels) is used. The anesthetic keeps you from feeling pain and, when given in injection form, also prevents the eye from moving around during the procedure or "seeing the surgery." An anesthesiologist usually monitors blood pressure, pulse, and other vital signs while the surgery is being performed.

## The Procedure

During the surgery, the eyelids are held open with a small metal instrument called a speculum. (Despite this, a patient does not see the operation as it happens.) A small opening is made through the conjunctiva to expose the sclera below. Once the sclera is visible, a small amount of cautery (coagulation of blood vessels using a heating instrument) is usually required because there are small blood vessels on the surface of the eye that bleed when the conjunctiva is opened and the superficial scleral tissue touched with any instrument. Within the sclera, a partial-thickness flap is made adjacent to and directly over the trabecular meshwork. The scleral flap is still attached to the eye and is not removed. The flap is simply lifted to reveal the drain below.

At this point in the surgery, I usually use Mitomycin-C (MMC), an antimetabolite (or antifibrosis) medication, to reduce postoperative scarring and bleb failure. Mitomycin-C was originally developed as an anticancer medication and is used topically in glaucoma surgery to prevent or reduce scarring. In essence, this drug prevents the body from satisfying its natural tendency to heal. Without this treatment, the body would want to "heal" the bleb too quickly. Excessive healing would cause premature closure of this newly created drain. For this reason, antimetabolite therapy was a major breakthrough in glaucoma surgery.

*MMC is applied before the eye itself is entered.* A small sponge, soaked with Mitomycin-C (with a concentration of 0.2 to 0.5 mg/mL), is applied to the surface of the eye either under or over the scleral flap. The conjunctiva is positioned above the flap and its edge is kept dry. During this time, a very small amount of MMC is being absorbed by the scleral bed, scleral flap, and overlying conjunctiva. On average, the sponge remains on the eye for thirty seconds to five minutes. MMC exposure time during the surgery will vary depending on the patient. More exposure to MMC is indicated in patients who are more likely to scar after surgery—those with a history of previous surgery, younger age, black, or glaucoma associated with inflammation. Less MMC time is used in older patients, those with a thin conjunctiva, or patients with no history of previous eye surgery. After the elapsed exposure time, the MMC-soaked sponge is removed and the surface of the eye is thoroughly irrigated with saline. Now that the MMC application is complete, the surgeon can safely enter the eye without getting MMC inside.

At this point, the eye is entered. A small portion of the trabecular meshwork that lies beneath the newly created flap is removed. Aqueous fluid begins to percolate through this drain. The surgeon can see the iris through this new drain. An iridectomy is performed so that the iris does not block the newly made drain. The scleral flap is then repositioned and closed with several sutures. (These sutures can be tied normally or made to be releasable. Releasable sutures are placed on the eye in a way that allows the surgeon to remove them—without cutting them—in the days to weeks after surgery.)

Because aqueous has been percolating out of the newly formed drain, the anterior chamber usually needs to be reinflated. A very tiny opening into the anterior chamber through the cornea is used to reinflate the front chamber of the eye (anterior chamber). This small opening is called a paracentesis. This reinflation is usually done with saline and/or air.

Sutures are placed on the flap until the flow of aqueous through the drain is acceptable to the surgeon. The number and position of these sutures will vary with each individual patient. The doctor tries to estimate the amount of aqueous that percolates through the drain. If too much aqueous comes through, more sutures are needed. If too little comes through, a suture may be loosened or removed.

Once the doctor has sutured the scleral flap into position over the drain and is confident that the aqueous flow is acceptable, the conjunctiva is closed over the flap with additional sutures. The wound is then checked to ensure that there are no leaks (to make sure that it is "watertight"). The speculum is removed. Antibiotic ointment is applied. A sterile patch and shield are placed over the eye and secured with tape. The patient is then discharged from the operating room.

## More on Antimetabolite (Antiscarring) Therapy

Antimetabolite therapy has increased the success rates of filtering surgery in those patients who are at greater risk of surgical failure (scarring of the drain). The first antimetabolite agent to be used (in conjunction with topical steroids) to reduce postoperative scarring and filter surgery failure was 5-fluorouracil (5-FU), not Mitomycin-C (MMC). Years ago, when 5-FU was introduced, injections of this medicine were given beneath the conjunctiva during the first two weeks after filtration surgery (two injections per day for the first week, followed by one injection daily for the second week). Though the routine was difficult to follow, the success rates for filtering surgery in eyes that were at high risk of failure (scarring) rose from 26 to 52 percent during three years of follow-up. Complications included corneal abrasions, bleb leaks, and bleb rupture.

Since those early days of 5-FU, the dosage and frequency of injections after filtering surgery were dramatically decreased. With fewer injections of 5-FU, the success rates appeared similar, but the complication rate decreased significantly.

With the introduction of Mitomycin-C and its use *during*

filtering surgery (not *after* surgery, as with 5-FU), the usage of 5-FU has dramatically *decreased*. MMC is approximately one hundred times more potent than 5-FU. The ability of MMC to be used in small doses for brief periods of time during the filtering surgery is a distinct advantage. (This is easier on both the patient *and* the glaucoma surgeon!) Complications related to MMC were found to be very similar to those with 5-FU, but those associated with MMC can occur later and be more serious. Today, 5-FU is used most frequently after a failing filter is revised in a procedure called the needling of the bleb, as discussed later in this chapter.

Not every filtering surgery requires the same amount of antimetabolite therapy. Some patients may not require MMC at all during surgery. Others will need a small exposure to MMC. Still others will require a more substantial exposure to MMC during the surgery. The doctor will consider each patient's unique risk factors for surgery failure, and the patient's likelihood of having scarring that would cause the filter to fail. Patients at greater risk of filter failure include:

- Patients with a history of previous eye surgery that may have scarred the conjunctiva.
- Patients who have already had glaucoma surgery that has failed.
- Patients with aphakia (absence of the natural lens of the eye, usually after cataract removal surgery, with no intraocular lens implant, or IOL).
- Patients who are young.
- Patients who are black.
- Patients with neovascular glaucoma (NVG).
- Patients with chronic inflammation such as iritis or uveitis.
- Patients who have used glaucoma medications over several or more years.
- Patients having simultaneous cataract surgery.

In this group of patients at higher risk of filter failure, the doctor will probably consider using Mitomycin-C during the surgery to improve the probability of success. If many risk factors for failure exist, the use of MMC is strongly considered, and the length of exposure to MMC during surgery may be increased accordingly.

*There is significant debate among glaucoma specialists as to just how Mitomycin-C should be used.* Some physicians use MMC very often and in practically all their filtering surgeries. Others argue that the risks associated with MMC outweigh the benefits. These risks include an increased incidence of hypotony (too-low IOP), since it can slow healing to such a degree that too much fluid leaves the eye. Hypotony can cause a significant reduction in vision (especially if the IOP is less than 8 mm Hg). The use of MMC can also result in a bleb that is very thin and leaky. Thin, leaky blebs may develop soon after surgery or months to years later. (Leaky blebs that develop months to years later are particularly worrisome to many glaucoma surgeons.) These thin, leaky blebs are predisposed to infection such as blebitis and endophthalmitis. For this reason, some argue that Mitomycin-C should never be used or should not be used in a patient who does not need a very low IOP. If hypotony does occur, it can often be managed through a bandage contact lens, surgical revision of the bleb, reduction in the use of topical anti-inflammatory agents, or other methods. However, even if hypotony is reversed, visual acuity may not be restored fully. In any case, the decision to use MMC is one that you should discuss with your doctor before surgery. Together, a decision that makes sense for you—as a unique individual—can be made.

Most of the literature supports the idea that antimetabolite therapy is very useful in glaucoma filtration surgery procedures, especially in the short term. However, long-term success is not as great as expected, and complications that occur long after surgery are serious and cannot be ignored. Despite this, many glaucoma specialists believe that MMC, when used judiciously, has made glaucoma filtering surgery more successful. For many glaucoma surgeons, MMC is used in practically all filtering surgeries. The amount used and exposure times are considered carefully and always individualized to obtain the best and safest results—in the short and the long term.

### How Successful Is Trabeculectomy?

Filtration surgery is currently the treatment of choice for most cases of glaucoma that cannot be controlled with medications and/or laser therapy. Studies of success are difficult to compare and summarize because they vary in terms of definition of *success*, glaucoma types, length of follow-up, surgical technique used, and patient demographics. Therefore, no simple statement regarding success can be made—except that there is a gradual decrease in the probability of successful IOP control over time. When a review of the many studies of long-term success after filtering surgery is conducted, the studies' success rates vary significantly. In one study, when *success* was defined as an IOP of less than 22 mm Hg without medication, success was reported as 60 to 98 percent. Long-term follow-up studies report success rates of 75 percent at ten years and 67 percent at fifteen years. Other studies reveal 90 percent success at five years, 67 percent at ten years, 48 percent at three years, and 40 percent at five years. Clearly, results vary tremendously.

The rate of cataract formation in patients with trabeculectomy is reported to be 22 to 38 percent.

### After Trabeculectomy Surgery

After filtering surgery, patients usually take a topical steroid eyedrop, a nonsteroidal eyedrop, a topical antibiotic eyedrop, and sometimes a medication that dilates the pupil. These medications help reduce inflammation and decrease the chances of developing a postoperative infection. The dilating drop is especially important if the postoperative IOP is lower than desired or the anterior chamber is shallow. These medications are used for several weeks (or more) after the surgery and are then gradually eliminated. During this postoperative period, some doctors give injections of 5-FU to further reduce scarring, especially if MMC was not used during surgery. Patients also need to wear an eye shield during sleep for several nights after surgery, and to limit their activities to a certain degree. The amount and type of allowable activity is unique to each individual and relates to how the eye looks and the level of IOP. (If the IOP is very low, the doctor may want activity levels to be more significantly reduced.)

A number of postoperative visits to the doctor are necessary after filtering surgery. The number and frequency depend on each patient's individual circumstances. Patients must always be seen on the first postoperative day and one week later, but in many cases the patient is examined every day, every other day, or every third day during the first week. It is important to understand that the IOP may fluctuate throughout the first few weeks after surgery, and, depending on the level and degree of fluctuation, it may need to be closely watched (with frequent follow-up exams).

Patients must also understand that during the surgery, sutures are used to secure the scleral flap that overlays the new drain. These sutures are crucial in controlling the amount of aqueous that flows through the surgically created drain. During the initial postoperative days to weeks, the scleral flap sutures can be cut—one at a time—using the argon or krypton laser. This is called laser suture lysis (LSL). With each suture that is cut, more aqueous is able to pass through the filter more easily, lowering the IOP. The doctor selectively cuts some or all of the sutures to guide the IOP to the desired level. (Most doctors routinely use postoperative LSL, since IOP is often higher than desired immediately after surgery. In general, glaucoma surgeons agree that it is easier to guide the IOP downward after filtering surgery then it is to raise it when too low.) Once cut, these flap sutures are left on the eye and do not usually need to be removed since they are covered by the conjunctiva. Also, after surgery, the doctor may need to gently massage the eye to encourage aqueous to flow through the drain and lower IOP. He or she may also instruct the patient to massage the eye to ensure that aqueous flows through the drain. Only under the direction of a physician should ocular massage be done.

### Complications of Trabeculectomy

During informed consent, you should become aware of all the common, significant complications of trabeculectomy—before you undergo the procedure. These complications include IOP that is too high or too low (hypotony), accelerated cataract development, hemorrhage (bleeding), infection (soon after surgery or months to years later), or the remote possibility of loss of vision.

You should also know that the bleb that will be created during surgery, though generally hidden from view beneath the upper lid, may be visible. In addition, during the postoperative period, the eyelid may be slightly droopy. In most cases, this is only temporary and will resolve in time (most postoperative droopy lids resolve well within six months). Sometimes, however, a bleb can create a *persistent* foreign-body sensation or discomfort.

A more serious, potential complication is endophthalmitis. This is an ocular infection that is a true medical emergency because it can permanently destroy the eye. The steps the doctor takes to avoid this postoperative infection include preoperative antibiotic drops, sterile technique, postoperative antibiotics, and close monitoring. *Since infection may occur despite all these precautions, do not hesitate to call the doctor if you experience extreme pain, redness, or light sensitivity after trabeculectomy—even if the glaucoma surgery was performed weeks, months, or years ago.*

### The Appearance and Feel of the Eye

After a trabeculectomy, the eye sometimes appears to be slightly red and can feel irritated. There may be tearing and a foreign-body sensation, as if something were in the eye. You may feel the sutures. These symptoms usually pass as the eye heals. The bleb is usually not visible since it is covered by the upper eyelid. After the eye has fully healed, the bleb is usually a pale, cystlike elevation that you can see when the upper lid is lifted.

### Vision After Trabeculectomy

Blurred vision immediately after trabeculectomy is common. Visual acuity typically returns to the preoperative level about one to three weeks after surgery. Vision may actually improve after the surgery if you are able to discontinue glaucoma medications that were impeding your ability to see clearly, such as pilocarpine. If significantly lowered IOP (especially less than 8 mm Hg) occurs, however, vision may worsen. Trabeculectomy may also hasten the development of cataracts or result in inflammation within the macula (macular edema), which will also impair vision. Macular edema is usually easily treated and remedied.

Your glasses may need to be changed after trabeculectomy. Contact lenses are only rarely worn after filtering surgery, because the bleb can easily be irritated or perforated by the lens or cause problems in lens fitting. Most importantly, the wearing of a contact lens after filtering surgery creates a greatly increased risk of vision-threatening infection (endophthalmitis).

## If a Trabeculectomy Fails

Trabeculectomies generally do not last forever, and their ability to control IOP generally decreases over time. Signs of a failing trabeculectomy are rising IOP and a bleb that is flattening.

If a trabeculectomy does fail, the doctor will consider adding one or more glaucoma medications (eyedrops). If medications fail to control the rising IOP, surgery would need to be performed again, and a new or revised bleb must be created.

Often, before medications are given or surgical revision is done in the operating room, the doctor may choose to do a brief (five- to fifteen-minute) procedure called a needling of the bleb. In this procedure, the failing bleb is anesthetized by injecting anesthetic medication (2 percent Xylocaine) underneath the conjunctiva near the bleb. Once numbed, a small needle (twenty-five- to thirty-gauge) is used to break superficial scar tissue that is blocking the flow of aqueous from the drain. This needling procedure can be done in conjunction with an injection of 5-fluorouracil under the conjunctiva to inhibit further scarring. Needling of the bleb is an effective and safe method of reviving a failing bleb. It can be done at the slit lamp or, preferably, under a microscope in a minor-procedure room. Unlike standard trabeculectomy surgery, a needling of the bleb need not be performed in the operating room.

## Which Should Be Used First: Medications or Filtration Surgery?

The important 2001 Collaborative Initial Glaucoma Treatment Study (CIGTS) compared the use of topical glaucoma medications to filtration surgery in patients with newly diagnosed primary open-angle glaucoma (POAG). The goal of the study was to determine if patients with newly diagnosed POAG did better if treated initially with medication or filtration surgery. Patients in the medication group were treated with a beta-blocker, with additional agents added if necessary. If medications failed to control IOP, patients underwent argon laser trabeculoplasty (ALT) and then, if that failed, trabeculectomy. Patients in the surgical treatment group underwent immediate trabeculectomy. If that treatment failed, they proceeded to ALT and then concluded with medications.

Results after five years showed that both groups had substantial reductions in IOP, with the surgical group having IOPs approximately 2 to 3 mm Hg lower than the medication group. In the first three years of the study, the surgical group had greater loss of visual field and visual acuity, but these differences disappeared by years four and five. Patients in the surgery group had more cataract surgeries than patients in the medication group. Both groups were satisfied with their treatments.

Researchers concluded that on the basis of study results to date, they did not recommend making any changes in the way open-angle glaucoma was currently being managed. *Results showed that initial treatment with either medication or trabeculectomy is effective in lowering IOP over a five-year follow-up.* In addition, both initial treatments were effective in stabilizing visual fields.

## DRAINAGE OR SHUNT DEVICES

Since the introduction of antimetabolite (antiscarring) therapy, the success associated with filtration surgery in high-risk glaucoma patients has increased. However, there is still a significant minority of glaucoma patients whose IOP cannot be controlled with traditional surgery. Aqueous shunts offer hope for these patients. Since the introduction of the Molteno implant in 1968, this alternative to traditional filtration surgery has given patients with refractory ("very difficult to successfully treat") glaucoma renewed hope of having their IOP controlled.

In general, aqueous shunts are reserved for patients who have failed traditional therapy or who are extremely unlikely to succeed with traditional therapy because of extensive conjunctival scarring. Aqueous shunts should be considered for patients with glaucoma who have uncontrolled IOP despite maximal medical therapy and whose conjunctiva is scarred extensively from previous failed filtration surgeries. Aqueous shunts can help control IOP in a variety of very difficult-to-treat glaucoma patients: those with refractory secondary glaucomas; patients who have had previous eye surgery or trauma associated with scarring; and those who have epithelial downgrowth (see glossary). Some glaucoma specialists consider the aqueous shunt to be the procedure of choice in neovascular glaucoma and some uveitic glaucomas (see chapter 4). In addition, some glaucoma specialists believe that aqueous shunts are less likely to result in endophthalmitis (a very serious, potentially blinding infection) because aqueous is shunted via a small tube toward a baseplate, which is located quite posteriorly on the sclera.

Clinical studies are now being performed to answer the question: Which procedure is better in a patient with poor prognosis (previous cataract surgery or failed trabeculectomies)—*trabeculectomy with MMC or an aqueous shunt?* The objective of one such study is to determine which of these two surgical interventions will provide the safest and most effective way to lower IOP in this group of difficult-to-manage, poor-surgical-prognosis glaucoma patients.

## What Is an Aqueous Shunt?

Aqueous shunts are implantable devices in which a small tube extends into the anterior chamber. The tube is connected to one or more plates, which are sutured to the surface of the eye. The most commonly used aqueous shunts are the Molteno implant, the Ahmed valved implant, and the Baerveldt implant.

The Molteno implants use a silicone tube without a valve. The tube is placed into the anterior chamber and guides aqueous to one or two plates sutured to the episclera, near the equator of the eye. As the eye heals, the plate becomes encapsulated by fibrous tissue and forms a bleb in a very posterior position (far back from the front of the eye).

One problem with some shunts is that the aqueous flows in an unrestricted fashion and lowers the IOP too much in the period right after surgery. This overfiltration may occur because the aqueous flows through the tube toward the plate without passing through a valve. IOP control using Molteno implants has improved through a design that uses two plates rather than one.

The Molteno implant is able to control IOP in 63 to 65 percent of aphakic and pseudophakic eyes with refractory glaucoma (when *success* is defined as an IOP of less than 22 mm Hg).

Recently, the Ahmed implant and the Baerveldt implant have gained in popularity. The Ahmed glaucoma valve implant (figure 31) has two distinct advantages over other aqueous shunts. Most important, it involves a valve system that helps prevent overfiltration and shallow or flat anterior chambers. Second, because it is positioned in only one quadrant of the eye, the surgeon does not need to manipulate or touch the eye's extraocular muscles. This type of valve implant has both a single-plate form and a double-plate system. Glaucoma specialists who use this implant often use the following guidelines for

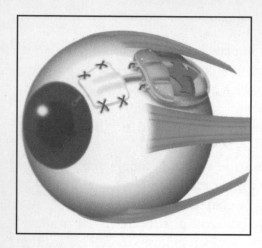

**Figure 31.** The Ahmed glaucoma valve implant. (Courtesy of H. Mateen Ahmed, M.D., New World Medical, Inc.)

choosing the patients to receive this device: patients who have failed traditional glaucoma filtration surgery; patients with active neovascular glaucoma; glaucoma associated with corneal transplants (penetrating keratoplasty, or PK); uveitic glaucomas; and aphakic infantile glaucomas. Overall, the Ahmed implant system has gained in popularity over recent years, becoming the *most commonly implanted* aqueous shunt in the world because of its simplicity of insertion and because its valved system significantly reduces the risk of overfiltration and hypotony (very low IOP).

The Baerveldt glaucoma implant involves a silicone tube that extends into the anterior chamber and is connected to a very thin plate that is attached to the eye. The plate is less than one millimeter thick—the thinnest glaucoma implant plate at this time. The silicone tube does not have a valve. The plates are kidney-shaped. Advantages of the Baerveldt implant are its large surface area (to improve drainage) and its ease of placement on the eye without disturbing the extraocular muscles.

Another popular valve is the Krupin valve shunt. The tube in this drainage device has a pressure-sensitive, one-way valve.

The valve system in the Krupin device helps guide the IOP to a range of 9–11 mm Hg.

## TRABECULOTOMY

Trabeculotomy is a surgical procedure for glaucoma in children.

This surgery is performed under general anesthesia. A small opening is made in the conjunctiva. This uncovers the sclera below, which lies immediately above the drain (trabecular meshwork). A partial-thickness flap is made in the sclera overlying the drain. A very small incision is made in the bed of the scleral flap, which is gradually deepened until the surgeon can see Schlemm's canal. A small metal instrument called a trabeculotome is gently passed into Schlemm's canal. The instrument is then gently rotated forward into the anterior chamber, breaking through the trabecular meshwork. This maneuver creates a passageway for aqueous to travel from the anterior chamber into Schlemm's canal in an unimpeded fashion. The instrument is removed and inserted into the other exposed portion of Schlemm's canal, and the maneuver is repeated. The scleral flap and conjunctiva are then closed with sutures.

## GONIOTOMY

Goniotomy is the surgery of choice in most cases of primary congenital glaucoma. It is also used in Sturge-Weber syndrome and other developmental glaucomas.

To perform this surgery safely, the surgeon must be able to visualize the anterior chamber. If the anterior chamber cannot be seen well, trabeculotomy is a preferred surgery.

In goniotomy, the surgeon places a clear magnifying lens (Barkan goniotomy lens) on the surface of the cornea. The eye is gently held in position with a pair of forceps. A small incision is made through the clear, peripheral cornea. A goniotomy knife is passed through this tiny corneal opening (paracentesis). An incision is made through the drain (trabecular meshwork). The opening is made in a circumferential way, across the four to five o'clock hours, opening one third or more of the drain and allowing aqueous to flow freely into Schlemm's canal and out of the eye. The tiny corneal incision is closed with a suture.

*Chapter 9*

# Surgery for Cataract and Glaucoma

A cataract is a clouding of the eye's natural lens. According to the National Eye Institute, nearly 20.5 million Americans age forty and older are affected by cataract. Cataract is the most commonly performed surgery in the Medicare population.

When a cataract causes reduced or poor vision (blur, glare, dimming of vision) that interferes with everyday life, it is usually time for surgical intervention. The most common procedure today is phacoemulsification, or phaco. During a routine phaco (pronounced *FAY-koh*), the doctor makes a tiny incision on the side of the cornea and inserts a very thin instrument into the eye. This thin, probelike instrument uses ultrasound waves from its tip to soften and break up the cloudy lens, which is then suctioned out in its entirety. (Interestingly, a cataract has the size and shape of one M&M candy. I will continue this analogy later as we discuss surgery in greater detail.) Once the eye's clouded lens is completely removed, a crystal-clear replacement intraocular lens (IOL) is inserted. The IOL is very flexible. During this surgery, the IOL is folded by the surgeon (or pre-folded by the manufacturer)—much like a very tiny taco—and then inserted through the same, tiny incision through which the cataract was removed. The IOL sits in the exact position that the old, cloudy lens once did. Stitches are typically not needed, because the little corneal incisions are self-sealing.

Since the incidence of both glaucoma *and* cataract increase as we age, it is not uncommon to find both conditions in the same patient simultaneously. If both require surgical treatment, the procedure becomes more complicated. Which should the doctor treat first? Should the two surgeries be combined?

## A BRIEF HISTORY

As recently as ten to fifteen years ago, combining cataract and glaucoma surgery was difficult because cataract surgery (before the days of phacoemulsification) required a large incision. Combining glaucoma surgery with such large-incision cataract surgery was often fraught with challenges. The popularity and success of combined cataract and glaucoma surgery increased with the advent of phacoemulsification, or small-incision surgery.

As microsurgical techniques improved, a new era in combined cataract-glaucoma surgery began. Using phacoemulsification, the success rates for a combined phacoemulsification plus trabeculectomy (phaco-trab) rivaled those for two-stage surgery—glaucoma filter surgery (trabeculectomy) and then cataract surgery at a later date, or vice versa.

The phaco-trab allows for a small incision, one closure, the use of antimetabolites, and the ability to use argon laser suture lysis (LSL) to guide postoperative intraocular pressure, or IOP, to the desired levels. Postoperative revision of the trabeculectomy is still easily performed either at the slit lamp or under the surgical microscope in a procedure called a needling of the bleb (see chapter 8).

## THE DECISION

When a patient presents with a visually significant cataract in the presence of glaucoma, the doctor (with the patient's assistance) must decide how to approach these coexisting problems. Often the doctor and patient choose from among the following three common options:

1. Cataract surgery alone.
2. Staged surgery: trabeculectomy followed by cataract surgery.
3. Combined cataract–glaucoma surgery (phaco-trab).

## CATARACT SURGERY ALONE

Cataract surgery alone (a routine phaco) provides a technically simple procedure with rapid postoperative visual recovery. It is a reasonable option when:

- There is a visually significant cataract and minimal, well-controlled glaucoma.
- A patient's glaucoma regimen consists of only one type of medication, and that medication is well tolerated.
- A patient has little or no glaucoma damage, central vision is not threatened, and there is unlikely to be further visual field loss if a postoperative IOP spike occurs.

In patients who require only one medication, the IOP after cataract surgery alone is often actually *reduced*. However, in the event that there is a postoperative IOP spike (sudden and significant rise), it is important to know that these patients are unlikely to develop further optic nerve damage and visual field loss as a result.

As with all decisions, though, it is important to consider the pros and cons before making a choice.

### Pros

A benefit to doing just cataract surgery is that this procedure alone *can* reduce IOP in some patients. In some patients with ocular hypertension (OHT—elevated IOP without glaucoma damage) or glaucoma patients who are well controlled with one medication, the IOP can actually be reduced following removal of the cataract. Another pro is that there is rapid post-operative recovery. Furthermore, trabeculectomy alone (performed later if required) is often more successful at controlling IOP than is combined cataract–glaucoma surgery.

### Cons

Cataract surgery alone could cause IOP to become more difficult to control. Also, there may be IOP spikes during the postoperative period. Certainly, if the optic nerve is fragile and could not tolerate a significant worsening of the IOP, cataract surgery alone is not a viable option.

### Technique

When possible, cataract surgery alone in a glaucoma patient should be done with a clear-cornea technique (the technique described at the beginning of this chapter). In a clear-cornea phacoemulsification, the conjunctiva is not incised. This preserves the conjunctiva, which may be needed for future glaucoma surgery such as a trabeculectomy.

# STAGED SURGERY: TRABECULECTOMY FOLLOWED BY CATARACT SURGERY (TWO SEPARATE PROCEDURES)

Doctors often consider this approach if:

- The patient has an advanced cataract. Significant inflammation could follow the surgery for this type of cataract and would limit the success of a simultaneous filtration surgery.
- The patient has a visually significant cataract and glaucoma that is poorly controlled or uncontrolled by the maximal tolerable medical regimen.
- The patient has advanced glaucomatous damage, and the optic nerve could be easily damaged by any postoperative IOP spike.

In these last two types of patients, glaucoma filtering surgery should be performed first so that IOP can be well controlled prior to performing the cataract surgery.

In patients who have ocular hypertension (OHT) or minimal glaucoma damage, trabeculectomy would usually be performed after cataract surgery if the IOP becomes uncontrolled in a significant way.

Studies have shown that when cataract surgery was followed by trabeculectomy, IOP remained controlled in 95 percent of patients. Other studies showed that filtering surgery followed by cataract surgery resulted in better long-term IOP control than was found in patients who underwent simultaneous cataract–glaucoma surgery (phaco-trab).

Overall, a staged surgical approach is often best for a patient with severe or poorly controlled glaucoma and for patients who have multiple risk factors for filtration failure.

It is always important for the doctor and patient to consider several additional factors. For instance, this approach exposes the patient to the possible complications associated with two separate surgeries. There is a longer recovery period as compared to the combined phaco-trab. In addition, there is the possibility of bleb failure after cataract surgery. Nevertheless, a staged surgical approach is still often best for a patient with severe or very poorly controlled glaucoma.

## COMBINED SURGERY (PHACO-TRAB)

Combined glaucoma–cataract surgery is well suited for:

- Patients with visually significant cataracts whose glaucoma control requires two or more medications (a key guideline that glaucoma surgeons often consider to a great degree).
- Patients with uncontrolled glaucoma that can be characterized as mild to moderate.
- Patients whose optic nerves are unable to tolerate postoperative IOP spikes.
- Patients who are poorly tolerant of their glaucoma medications.
- Patients unable to tolerate two separate surgeries.

One clear advantage to the phaco-trab is that the patient only has to undergo one single surgery for each eye. Phaco-trab surgery is associated with an excellent success rate and can protect the patient's optic nerve against postoperative IOP spikes. Disadvantages include the fact that this is a technically more difficult surgery to perform, and the IOP control may not be as good as with trabeculectomy alone.

Overall, phaco-trab is an effective, well-tolerated surgery with a visual recovery that is usually only a few days longer than the recovery period associated with cataract surgery alone.

### Phaco-Trab: The Surgical Procedure

The combined phaco-trab can be performed in a variety of ways. Some surgeons prefer to remove the cataract and insert the implant through a clear corneal incision, then choose a separate site to perform a standard trabeculectomy. An equally acceptable choice is to perform both procedures through one small incision. Both methods provide excellent postoperative results. Both procedures allow for the use of Mitomycin-C (MMC) and will allow for postoperative argon laser suture lysis. However, when a single site is chosen, the operative time is generally less than with two-site surgery. Single-site surgery also means that only one area of the eye is touched. Single-site phaco-trab is generally my procedure of choice when a phaco-trab is indicated, but other surgeons prefer the two-site method.

In phaco-trab surgery, informed consent is obtained after the risks and benefits of the surgery are discussed with the patient. Preoperative medications and precautions are performed just as for the patient undergoing standard filtering surgery (trabeculectomy) alone. Preoperatively, the patient uses an antibiotic eye drop (for instance, a fourth-generation fluoroquinolone such as Vigamox or Zymar) and a nonsteroidal anti-inflammatory eyedrop (such as Acular) four times per day for the three days prior to surgery.

Upon arrival at the ambulatory surgery center, dilating eyedrops are given several times. (Additional nonsteroidal anti-inflammatory drops, such as Acular or Voltaren, and antibiotic eyedrops are also given.) Prior to entering the operating room, additional dilating medications are usually given to ensure adequate dilation of the pupil. Following this, 2 percent Xylocaine jelly (lidocaine HCL) is applied to help numb the eye. (Though it's not always needed, it is at this point that an injection of anesthetic can be given around or near the eye to numb it and reduce eye movement during surgery.)

In the operating room, a small wire instrument called a speculum holds the eyelids open. (Despite this, the patient is unable to see the surgery taking place.) A small incision is made in the conjunctiva to reveal the scleral tissue below. When this opening is made, often a small amount of bleeding is seen. Minimal cautery controls this bleeding and is performed at this time. *Prior* to entering the eye, Mitomycin-C (MMC) is applied using a small sponge. The sponge is held in place for a period of time unique to each individual patient, but averaging approximately thirty seconds to five minutes. Copious irrigation with saline solution rinses all residual MMC from the eye surface after the specified interval has elapsed.

After Mitomycin is used, a small incision measuring approximately 2.75 millimeters in length is made in the sclera. A tunneled incision is then made into the sclera and peripheral cornea beginning at that small scleral incision site. The anterior chamber is filled with 1 percent nonpreserved lidocaine solution, followed by a viscoelastic material such as Viscoat or Healon. These materials are injected into the anterior chamber via a tiny (less than one millimeter) incision in the cornea, approximately three clock hours away from the main incision. Following this, the eye is entered using a sharp, pointed blade that passes through the tunneled incision into the anterior chamber.

At this point, the doctor will be looking carefully at the size of the patient's pupil. Often, in glaucoma—especially in patients with pseudoexfoliation, patients who have been on long-term glaucoma medications (particularly pilocarpine), or patients who have had episodes of inflammation within the anterior chamber—pupillary dilation is poor. To safely perform the cataract surgery, the pupil must be adequately dilated. If the pupil is poorly dilated, the doctor will stretch it open using fine hooks in a gentle stretching maneuver. Once the pupil is of adequate size, the surgery continues.

A bent thirty-gauge needle is used to make a small opening in the anterior capsule (very much like the candy coating shell of the M&M) of the lens, and a small circular portion of the capsule is removed using forceps. A fine, pencil-shaped instrument with ultrasound at its very tip is placed into the eye, and the cataract lens (the chocolate inside of the M&M) is broken into small pieces and suctioned from the eye, keeping the capsular bag or sac of the lens (the M&M shell) intact. Once all the lens material has been removed, the crystal-clear folded intraocular lens is inserted via the tiny, tunneled incision into the capsular bag from which the cataract was just removed.

The doctor's attention now turns to the trabeculectomy portion of the surgery. Just beneath the opening of the scleral tunnel lies the trabecular meshwork (drain). A small portion of this meshwork is removed, and aqueous is seen to easily percolate through. An iridectomy (surgical removal of a piece of iris tissue) is usually performed using small scissors. The doctor then uses sutures to close the newly formed drain. Repeatedly, the doctor will check the newly formed drain to evaluate the aqueous flow. Once satisfied that the amount of aqueous flowing through the drain is appropriate, the doctor will reposition the conjunctiva into its normal position and close it with several sutures. All remaining Healon and Viscoat are removed from the eye. Filtration is then checked again as the anterior chamber is inflated with saline. The surgeon will check thoroughly for leaks, confirming that the aqueous that flows through the newly created drain will flow out of it and under the conjunctiva—and stay there. (No leaks!)

The speculum is then removed, and antibiotics are applied to the eye. At this point, some doctors inject a small amount of antibiotic and/or steroid beneath the conjunctiva. This depends on the individual surgeon's preference. (Doctors still debate whether this step is necessary or not.) This is followed by the placement of a patch and shield. The patient is then discharged from the operating room and observed in the recovery area for approximately one hour.

## The Challenge of Cataract Surgery in the Presence of Glaucoma

Phacoemulsification in patients with glaucoma can be challenging for several reasons. Often, glaucoma patients' pupils will not adequately dilate, especially when there is pseudoexfoliation, if patients have been on chronic miotic therapy (with, say, pilocarpine), or if there is a history of inflammation in the anterior chamber causing adhesions (synechiae) in the eyes and lens. The surgeon must be extremely skilled in the removal of a cataract in the presence of a small pupil. A pupil can be dilated with a manual technique prior to removing the cataract. This is often done using two small instruments that gently stretch the pupil open. Pupillary dilation prior to phacoemulsification must be done gently and minimally. If the pupil is stretched too far, it may permanently remain large and dilated, producing postoperative glare and blur. (Unfortunately, even with the gentlest technique, this may occur.)

My preferred method to enlarge a small pupil is to use the bimanual (two-handed) technique of stretching with two Kuglen iris hooks. These hooks stretch the pupil just enough to safely enlarge it and make it so that there is adequate visualization to safely remove the cataract. With this technique of manual stretching, the postoperative pupil is generally round, of good size, and of good mobility. There is less inflammation, less bleeding, and the edges of the implant are well covered.

# PSEUDOEXFOLIATION AND CATARACT

If you have pseudoexfoliation (exfoliation syndrome or exfoliative glaucoma) and cataract, you will present an exceptional challenge for your surgeon. The natural lens of the eye is held in place by thousands of small fibers called zonules. As we saw in chapter 4, patients with pseudoexfoliation often have zonular laxity (weakening) in addition to a poorly dilating pupil. This can be problematic during cataract surgery. When the phaco ultrasound instrument is used to break up the lens, the lens must remain firmly anchored in position. This anchoring of the eye's natural lens in its position is the job of the zonules. When the zonules that hold the lens in place are weak or broken, as is often the case in pseudoexfoliation, the surgeon must take extra care to ensure that no further damage to the zonules occurs and that the capsular bag remains completely intact throughout the surgery. Gentle manipulation of the cataract lens and awareness of the zonular laxity *at all times during the surgery* are crucial for a successful and uncomplicated outcome to the procedure. In addition, a capsular tension ring (chapter 14) may be required to stabilize the capsule.

If you have pseudoexfoliation and you begin to develop a visually significant cataract, you should talk to your doctor about proceeding to surgery *sooner rather than later*. As a cataract develops and matures, it becomes not only thicker (in the same way that the trunk of a tree adds rings), but also harder. A thicker, harder lens requires more phaco ultrasound energy to break it into pieces when it is being removed. When pseudoexfoliation is present, it is far safer to perform cataract surgery earlier, when less phaco energy is required—especially if there is zonular laxity and/or damage. The concept of waiting until a cataract is "ripe" does not apply in today's phaco surgery—especially if there is pseudoexfoliation present.

# Chapter 10

# Nutrition and Eye Health

Up to this point, this book has discussed traditional medical treatments such as eyedrops and surgery. Recently, however, some patients and health care providers have begun to use nontraditional therapies such as vitamins, herbal remedies, acupuncture, and exercise to fight glaucoma. These types of treatment can all be categorized as complementary and alternative medicine (CAM). Approximately 54 out of 1,000 glaucoma patients (5 percent) use some sort of CAM treatment, but that number is growing rapidly.

In this chapter, I will discuss nutrition and herbal supplements as possible treatments for glaucoma and the importance of weight control. I will describe the state of our knowledge to date and explain how you can incorporate this information into your everyday lifestyle. Chapter 11 will cover the remaining CAM therapies.

The importance of nutrition in protecting you from serious illnesses such as cardiovascular disease, hypertension, osteoporosis, and certain cancers has been well documented. Chances are, you have heard a lot—both from your doctors and from the media—about the kinds of foods you should be eating to protect your heart, blood vessels, bones, colon, and other organs. But did you realize that certain foods and supplements might also protect your eyes? A growing body of clinical evidence suggests that we may be able to improve the overall health of our eyes and reduce the impact of serious eye disorders by following specific nutritional guidelines.

Before you even consider incorporating nutritional therapy into your treatment regimen, it is important to consult your internist. You must make sure that any alternative treatment you are considering will not interfere with medications you are already taking or any general health problems you may have. *It is also key that your doctors be kept abreast of any herbal or other nutritional therapies you try.* Nutritional supplements and vitamins may contribute to healthier eyes, but they may also pose possible health risks. (Many of their beneficial and harmful effects may not be known at this time.)

## DISEASE-FIGHTING PROPERTIES OF PLANT FOODS

One of the reasons that plant foods such as fruits, vegetables, and grains are so good for us is that they are rich in disease-fighting compounds. Some of these compounds are called antioxidants. Antioxidants help neutralize the damage caused by free radicals, which are substances generated by our bodies during the normal process of metabolism. Free radicals may also result from poor lifestyle choices such as exposure to cigarette smoke, alcohol, environmental toxins, or sunlight.

Antioxidants include vitamin C, vitamin E, and a group of substances called carotenoids. Carotenoids are the pigments that are synthesized by plants. Beta-carotene (which is converted into vitamin A in your body) is probably the best-known carotenoid; it is found in red, orange, and yellow fruits and vegetables (sweet potatoes, apricots, cantaloupes, carrots, red and yellow peppers) and dark green leafy vegetables (spinach, kale, collard greens—the darker, the better). Some carotenoids are converted to vitamin A in our bodies. Vitamin E is found in vegetable oil, nuts, and seeds, while vitamin C is abundant in fruits and vegetables such as oranges, grapefruit, red pepper, and broccoli.

There are literally hundreds of different carotenoids in foods—and that is only one category of the many disease-fighting substances found in fruits and vegetables. For that reason, it is difficult to separate out exactly which individual antioxidant is responsible for protecting us from which disease. It is probably the combination of vitamins, minerals, antioxidants, and other compounds in nutrients that makes a plant-based diet so effective in reducing the risk of cardiovascular disease, stroke, and certain cancers.

A number of landmark studies have recently shown that what we eat also affects the health of our eyes.

### Age-Related Eye Disease Study (AREDS)

Age-related macular degeneration (ARMD) is a leading cause of visual impairment and blindness in the United States. It is a condition in which the central area of the retina, the macula, degenerates. Macular degeneration, which mainly affects older individuals, results in an irreversible loss of central vision. There is only very limited treatment for ARMD.

A number of animal and observational studies have suggested that antioxidants and the trace elements zinc and selenium might be associated with a reduced risk of ARMD (as well as a reduced risk for cataract development). Based on these results and the results of a small clinical trial suggesting that zinc supplementation could reduce vision loss, the National Eye Institute (NEI) of the National Institutes of Health (NIH) sponsored the Age-Related Eye Disease Study.

The two main purposes of the AREDS were to evaluate the effects of high doses of antioxidants and zinc on the progression of ARMD and vision loss and to evaluate the effects of high doses of antioxidants on the development and progression of cataract and vision loss. The antioxidant formula used was: 500 milligrams vitamin C, 400 International Units vitamin E, 15 milligrams beta-carotene, 80 milligrams zinc as zinc oxide, and 2 milligrams copper as cupric oxide.

Results showed that people at high risk for developing advanced ARMD (those with intermediate ARMD and those with advanced ARMD in one eye) reduced their chances of progressing to advanced ARMD by 25 percent when they took antioxidants plus zinc. In this group, antioxidants plus zinc also reduced the risk of central vision loss by 19 percent. People at high risk for developing advanced ARMD treated with zinc alone reduced their risk of developing ARMD by 21 percent and their risk of vision loss by 11 percent. Participants who were treated with antioxidants alone reduced their risk of developing advanced ARMD by approximately 17 percent and their risk of vision loss by approximately 10 percent. These same nutrients had no effect on the development of cataract.

Studies have shown that individuals who consume diets high in leafy green vegetables have a lower risk of developing ARMD. However, the level of nutrients consumed by participants in AREDS would be difficult to achieve from food alone.

Although AREDS did not assess the effect of antioxidants or zinc on intraocular pressure (IOP) or optic nerve damage in glaucoma, it does establish a relationship between the intake of certain nutrients and the condition of the eye—at least in terms of ARMD. Until we know more, it would be wise for all glaucoma patients—as well as anyone at risk for glaucoma—to follow a diet that is rich in dark, leafy green vegetables.

Do the macula and glaucoma relate to each other? *Yes.* Does knowledge of the macula help us know more about glaucoma? *Yes?*

Glaucoma is a group of disorders characterized by a final common pathway: ganglion cell death. This ganglion cell loss manifests itself as a loss of axons and cupping of the optic nerve head. Remarkably, the majority of the eye's entire population of retinal ganglion cells lies within the macula.

Glaucoma doctors acknowledge the importance of studying the macula and its wealth of ganglion cells, and are developing ways to correlate changes in the macula with changes related to glaucoma, such as the retinal thickness analyzer (RTA), and optical coherence tomography (OCT); you will learn more about this in chapter 13. Clearly, nutrition and lifestyle choices that have a proven positive effect on the macula could possibly relate to glaucoma as well. But only further research can confirm this.

### Lutein and Zeaxanthin

Lutein and zeaxanthin, antioxidants that belong to the carotenoid family of antioxidants, are both concentrated in the retina and lens of the eye.

A number of studies that look at disease trends in various populations have indicated that people who ate diets high in lutein-containing foods had a lower incidence of certain eye diseases. For instance, a study supported by the National Eye Institute showed that individuals who ate carotenoid-rich leafy, green vegetables such as collard greens, kale, and spinach had a lower risk of developing ARMD. Other data showed a reduced incidence of cataract surgery in women with diets high in lutein and zeaxanthin. These data were confirmed in numerous additional studies, although some studies have failed to verify the association. The NEI is currently conducting further research to evaluate this relationship.

Lutein and zeaxanthin are the only carotenoids that become concentrated within the macula. These high levels within the macula protect the retina by reducing free radical damage and absorbing damaging blue light rays. In fact, among antioxidant nutrients, lutein and zeaxanthin appear to be the most effective in protecting the health of the eye. Researchers believe that the antioxidant effect of these nutrients provides significant protection against the harmful rays of the sun.

Foods high in lutein are egg yolk, kale, spinach, broccoli, corn, romaine lettuce, peas, zucchini, and other colorful fruits and vegetables. Zeaxanthin is found in many of the same foods as lutein, but foods such as orange juice, oranges, and corn contain more zeaxanthin than lutein. (Ironically, the carrots we all ate as children because we thought they were "good for our eyes" do not contain lutein and zeaxanthin . . . although they do contain beta-carotene, which is an antioxidant—but one that is *not* usually found in the eye.)

Again, there are no data linking lutein and zeaxanthin to a beneficial effect on glaucoma. But eating fruits and vegetables is always a good idea. If you have glaucoma, it is important to keep your eyes (and your body) as healthy as possible overall. In addition, many experts believe that researchers have yet to discover all the potential benefits of good nutrition for preserving our vision.

### Wine

One early study suggested that people who drank wine in moderation might be less likely to develop ARMD. However, the NEI believed that no recommendation could be made on the basis of this single study. Moreover, later studies have not supported these findings. Wine may be beneficial to the heart, but as yet there is no documented proof that it helps keep your eyes healthy. If the relationship does hold true, however, it may also apply to the skins of red grapes—not just red wine.

## Vitamin C

Researchers have found that there are high concentrations of vitamin C in the aqueous humor, vitreous (twenty-five times our serum level), and retina (one hundred times our serum level). Intravenous vitamin C is effective in lowering IOP, but the effect was not always seen with the oral form of vitamin C, even in high doses. Several studies found that vitamin C in very large doses (20 grams daily or higher) successfully reduced IOP. The mechanism of this is unknown. These same researchers acknowledge that vitamin C is *not* a cure for glaucoma, and that as soon as the vitamin C doses are reduced, IOP rises.

## Vitamin E

The antioxidant properties of vitamin E help protect the eye and lens. In some research, vitamin E added to regular glaucoma medication was shown to improve visual fields in a majority of patients studied. Other researchers have not confirmed this finding, however.

Future research will examine the possible role of vitamin E in preventing glaucoma optic neuropathy now that a study done at Johns Hopkins has shown that vitamin E (in a dose of 46.5 milligrams per day) reduces the risk of developing the neurodegenerative Alzheimer's disease by 26 percent.

## Fish Oil (Omega-3 Fatty Acids)

Individuals with a high intake of omega-3 fatty acids (found in fish and fish oil) appear to have a lower incidence of certain eye diseases. In one study, approximately forty-three thousand women and thirty thousand men were followed for ten to twelve years. At the end of that time, individuals who had consumed more than four servings of fish per week had a 35 percent lower risk of ARMD than those consuming three or fewer servings. In addition, intake of linolenic acid (found in canola oil) and total fat intake were both associated with a higher risk of ARMD. *Again, there were no data regarding glaucoma.* However, it has been suggested that fish oil may reduce IOP and be relevant to glaucoma because of its protective effect on the macula.

Several studies have shown that the Inuit, who have a high intake of omega-3 (as found in fish and unrefined fish oils), have a very low incidence of open-angle glaucoma. Other studies in animals show that fish oil can lower IOP.

Good sources of omega-3 are cold-water fish such as salmon, cod, and mackerel, black currant seed oil, and flaxseed oil. A diet that includes fish three or more times per week seems ideal.

### Chromium

The American diet often consists of very highly processed foods. Unfortunately, the refining process causes food to lose chromium (among other nutrients). It is estimated that 90 percent of all Americans' diets are low in chromium. Low levels of dietary chromium are believed to be a risk factor for increased IOP.

Studies show that chromium affects the insulin receptor within the eye, and low levels of chromium are strongly associated with glaucoma. The details of this association and the relation between chromium and glaucoma are not yet known, but chromium's role in protecting the small blood vessels within the eye may be important.

Dietary sources of chromium include brewer's yeast, lean meats, cheeses, pork kidney, whole-grain bread and cereals, molasses, spices, and bran cereals. On the other hand, vegetables, fruits, and highly-refined and processed foods (except processed meats) all contain low levels of chromium.

### Miscellaneous Nutrients

Other nutrients that have been hypothesized to have a positive effect on glaucoma—because of a *possible* neuroprotective action or other properties—include lipoic acid, vitamin $B_{12}$, magnesium, glucosamine, carnitine, selenium, coenzyme Q10, and folic acid. To date, however, there is no clinical proof to support these hypotheses.

## HERBS

In the United States, herbs are not subject to the same rigorous testing and approval process by the Food and Drug Administration (FDA) that pharmaceutical products are. However, herbs are in wide use—both in the U.S. and abroad. For this reason, many have been widely studied. With regard to their effects on health, Commission E, a German regulatory agency roughly equivalent to our FDA, has conducted extensive studies of many herbal products. Based on its review of the literature, Commission E pronounces substances either "approved" or "unapproved" for use. Be aware, though, that these reviews may not involve the same rigorous standards required by our FDA.

You should also bear in mind that the herbs you see on the shelves of your supermarkets or pharmacies, or that you purchase on the Internet, have not been manufactured according to FDA standards. They may not contain the amount of active ingredients stated on the label, or they may not dissolve completely once they are ingested.

My advice with herbs is the same as my advice with all CAM therapies: Work with your doctor. If your doctor advises you to take an herbal preparation, he or she will probably also be able to recommend a reliable manufacturer. You can also ask your pharmacist to recommend the highest-quality products.

### Ginkgo Biloba

The fact that ginkgo biloba is believed to improve central and peripheral blood flow, reduce vasospasm (spasm of the blood vessels), reduce serum viscosity, and have antioxidant activity raises the possibility that this herb may be a potential antiglaucoma therapy.

Ginkgo biloba extract is created from the dried leaves of the ginkgo tree. It has been shown to relax blood vessels and improve blood supply to the brain. While many believe that ginkgo biloba is effective in treating glaucoma, this has not yet been proven. It is also widely theorized that ginkgo biloba improves memory, reduces the chances of developing dementia (or slowing its progression), improves peripheral vascular circulation, reduces the symptoms of asthma and bronchitis, and improves sexual functioning. Commission E states that its clinical uses include the treatment of dementia where the following symptoms are present: memory deficits, depression, dizziness, tinnitus (ringing in the ear), and headaches. It also increases pain-free walking in patients with peripheral arterial occlusive disease. It can be used in the treatment of vertigo and tinnitus of vascular origin. A side effect of ginkgo biloba is that it can possibly lead to intestinal upsets, headaches, or allergic skin reactions. Spontaneous bleeding has also been reported, and gingko may interact with anticoagulant and antiplatelet agents. For that reason, ginkgo biloba should not be taken in conjunction with anticoagulant therapy such as Coumadin. Recommended dosages are 120 to 240 mg spread out over two or three doses throughout the day.


### Bilberry

Bilberry is a dried fruit from the Ericaceae family. It contains tannins (such as those found in tea and red wine) as well as other forms of antioxidants. Bilberry is reported to strengthen blood vessels and improve the eye's ability to see in dim light (thereby enhancing night vision). There are anecdotal, unsubstantiated reports that bilberry was used by World War II pilots to enhance night vision. Bilberry has no proven effect on IOP or visual field. According to Commission E, bilberry is mainly recommended for acute diarrhea and mild inflammation of the mouth and throat. Dosage is usually 40 to 60 milligrams per day.


### Pasqueflower

The pasqueflower herb consists of the dried parts of *Anemone pulsatilla*. It is not approved for use by Commission E, but its claimed applications are for diseases of the genital organs, inflammatory and infectious diseases of the skin and mucosa, and disorders of the gastrointestinal and urinary tracts. It is also reported to help relieve eye inflammation related to glaucoma and retinal problems associated with cataract; however, this remains unproven. There are several risks associated with the use of pasqueflower. Internal use in high dosages can result in irritation to the kidneys and urinary tract. Topical use can produce severe irritation on the skin and mucosa with itching, rash, and pustule. Pasqueflower is absolutely contraindicated in pregnancy.

## Melatonin and Aspirin

Both of these agents have been hypothesized to affect IOP; however, this has not been confirmed by clinical studies.


# WEIGHT CONTROL

Obesity is associated with poor overall health. If you are overweight, you are more likely to develop cardiovascular disease, diabetes, hypertension, and certain cancers. And you may be putting yourself at additional risk for glaucoma. To lose weight, you need to consume fewer calories than your body burns. The actual number of calories it will take to do that will depend on your frame, your activity level, your muscle mass, your age, and your genes.

Losing one pound of fat requires a thirty-five-hundred-calorie deficit over time. There are two ways to accomplish this: You can reduce the number of calories you eat, and/or you can increase your activity level to burn more calories. The best way to lose weight is to do both. In the next chapter, I will talk about exercise. For now, I will discuss losing weight by changing your eating habits.

Reducing the calories you eat doesn't always mean eating less. Your first step should be *changing* the foods you eat. Increasing your consumption of fruits, vegetables, and whole grains should help you naturally cut calories without entering into starvation mode. Cutting fat is an especially efficient way of cutting calories, since one fat gram is worth nine calories (compared to four calories each for protein and carbohydrates). For instance, baking your chicken instead of frying it (and taking the skin off for good measure) is a relatively simple way to lighten up.

Don't try to lose weight too quickly. Weight lost from fad diets usually comes right back as soon as you begin eating normally again. The best advice I can give you is to aim for a slow, steady weight loss of half a pound to one pound per week, and develop an eating plan you can stick with throughout your lifetime—under the supervision and guidance of your internist. (That is a must!)

If you've tried your best to improve your diet and increase your exercise but the weight isn't coming off, you may have an undiagnosed medical problem—such as a thyroid disorder—that is making it difficult for you to lose weight. Clearly, weight control is best managed with your internist's help!

# Chapter 11

# Exercise, Stress Reduction, Lifestyle, and Glaucoma

In 1997, Americans spent twenty-seven billion dollars on various complementary and alternative (CAM) treatments. That figure is relevant to us, since some 5 percent of all glaucoma patients have been estimated to use a complementary and alternative treatment of some sort.

In the previous chapter, I discussed the roles of vitamins, herbs, general nutrition, and weight reduction. Here, I will describe the role of exercise in glaucoma treatment and discuss therapies even less mainstream, such as meditation and acupuncture. It is important to understand all these "treatments," because some of them may be *harmful* while others can contribute to the overall health of your eyes.

## SMOKING

One lifestyle choice that is known to elevate intraocular pressure (IOP) is smoking. Under your doctor's supervision, stop smoking! Several important studies have linked current smoking and elevated IOP. Research has shown that nicotine causes circulatory changes within the body, particularly vasospasm (spasm of the blood vessels) in small vessels. It is believed that nicotine may trigger the constriction of the episcleral veins. This inhibits the outflow of aqueous from the trabecular meshwork, and an elevation of IOP results.

## EXERCISE

In addition to being good for your heart, blood vessels, bones, and just about every other part of your body, exercise is also good for your eyes. Aerobic exercise (exercise that increases your heart rate and respiratory rate, such as brisk walking, bicycling, jogging), performed on a regular basis, has been documented to lower IOP. Some studies show that regular exercise can reduce IOP by an average of 20 percent. Exercise may also improve blood flow to the retina and optic nerve. Here is an incentive to make exercise a permanent part of your daily routine: Once the aerobic exercise ceases, IOP returns to its previous levels.

By exercising regularly, you will also be protecting yourself from a variety of other unhealthy conditions—many of them chronic diseases such as diabetes, hypertension, and certain cancers. In fact, after reviewing the medical literature, the authors of a study that appeared in *Journal of Applied Physiology* concluded that ". . . with the possible exception of diet modification, we know of no single intervention with greater promise than physical exercise to reduce the risk of virtually all chronic diseases simultaneously."

Here are just some of the diseases and conditions associated with sedentary living:

• Type 2 diabetes.
• Cardiovascular disease.

- Hypertension.
- High cholesterol.
- Breast and colon cancers.
- Osteoporosis.

## What to Do?

First, take a positive and hope-filled approach to an exercise regimen. Exercise should be viewed as a prescription to be enjoyed, not endured. Your goal in planning an exercise program should be to select activities that you will enjoy doing. Think of each of your workouts as your own special time—a time you need and deserve to unwind and recover from the stresses of your day. Otherwise, you will have a hard time sticking to your plan.

To increase your general activity level, begin with small steps. Take the stairs instead of the elevator, and park at the far end of the lot instead of at the front. Do you live within walking distance of a store or mall? Start doing some of your errands on foot. Take a stroll to visit a friend instead of picking up the phone. Plant a garden. Wash your car. If the weather is bad, drive to your local shopping mall and log a few laps as you window-shop. Put on some music and dance. Ride a bicycle. Go for a swim.

To make working out even more fun, convince a friend or partner to join you. That will also make it more difficult for you to skip a day.

If you are interested in beginning a more formal exercise program, it should include each of these elements: aerobic, strength, flexibility, and balance/stability training. Naturally, any exercise program should involve the guidance of your internist.

## Aerobic Training

Aerobics, or endurance exercises, such as walking, running, biking, and dancing, cause your heart rate to increase for an extended period of time. Since your heart is a muscle, causing it to work harder strengthens it. Aerobic exercises also strengthen your lungs and circulatory system and help blood sugar. Not only will this enhance your health and build stamina, but it will also burn calories.

Whenever you move your body faster than usual to perform any aerobic exercise, your heart begins to beat faster (your pulse increases), and your breathing becomes heavier (your respiratory rate increases). As you increase your activity level, the muscles in your body require increased amounts of blood and oxygen as nourishment. The more intense your activity, the faster your heart will beat, and the more deeply you will breathe. But there is no need for you to spend your entire workout gasping and gulping for air. Moderate exercise can be just as good for you as more vigorous exercise, like running.

To reduce your IOP, you should spend about thirty minutes doing aerobic exercise at least four days a week. If you haven't been exercising lately, it will take some time to work up to thirty minutes of activity. Add as little as five minutes at a time until you get there. Start out each session slowly so your body has a chance to warm up.

Don't feel as though you have to go all-out for the full thirty minutes of each exercise session. In general, there is a target heart rate zone for each of us, and as long as your heart rate falls within that zone, your health will benefit. To calculate your target heart rate, subtract your age from the number 220. That number, in beats per minute (bpm), is your maximum heart rate. Your target zone is generally 50 to 80 percent of that number. For instance, if you are a fifty-year-old woman, your maximum heart rate is 170 bpm. Your target heart rate zone is 50 to 80 percent of that, or 85 to 136 bpm. Where you should aim within that zone depends on your health and fitness level. Your internist can help out by reviewing your exercise plans with you.

If you work out in a gym, you will find that many tread-mills, exercise bikes, and other pieces of equipment now come with heart rate monitors. Portable heart rate monitors that fit around your chest can also be purchased at sporting goods stores. But it won't cost you a cent to take a moment out of your workout to measure your own pulse. The carotid pulse should be easy for you to find. Place two fingers on one side of your neck, below your chin bone and almost directly under your ear. You should feel the throbbing of your pulse. Or you can check the pulse on the inside of your wrist, if you find that easier. Either way, count the beats for ten seconds, multiply by six, and you will know your heartbeats per minute. If you can do this safely while exercising, it will give you the most accurate measure. Otherwise, take your reading immediately upon stopping, before your body has had a chance to cool down.

Even without taking your pulse, you should be able to tell if your heart is beating too fast. A general rule of thumb is that if you are breathing too hard to talk, you should slow down. But if you can sing without any problem, you probably are not exercising hard enough.

### Strength Training

As we age, we all lose muscle mass and our bones weaken. This is especially true for women. Not only does this increase the likelihood of weight gain, but it also makes us physically weaker. Strength training can help prevent this. Except in cases where a patient has very advanced glaucoma-related nerve damage, I allow weight training, although I discourage extreme amounts of weight.

Even small increases in muscle mass can yield great improvements in our ability to function and lead independent lives as we grow older. Another especially important benefit of strength exercises is that they can help prevent osteoporosis. Resistance training can also reduce your risk of cardiovascular disease. If you have Type 2 diabetes, this type of exercise can help improve your glucose tolerance and insulin sensitivity.

In general, free weights and ankle weights are inexpensive, and they do not take up much room in your house. You can also build muscle through resistance training with elastic bands (available at sporting goods stores). If you prefer a gym setting, you will probably have a greater choice of equipment. Your local Y or community center may also have a good workout facility, and you may prefer the atmosphere. One benefit of a gym or your local Y is that there will be instructors present to make sure that you are doing the exercises correctly. Some professional guidance, at least at the beginning, can help ensure that you are using the proper form for your workout. A trainer can show you how to prevent injuries and help you get the maximum benefit from your workout.

If you decide to start strength training on your own, here are some general guidelines:

- Aim for twice a week. Do not exercise the same muscle group two days in a row.
- Start with a weight you can lift for a minimum of eight repetitions (reps). If you can comfortably lift it for fifteen reps, increase the amount of weight you use for your next workout. Increase gradually.
- Perform each exercise two to three times (sets).
- Breathe out when you perform the hard part of the exercise (lifting or pushing). Breathe in on the easy part. Do not hold your breath.
- Perform the exercises smoothly. Lift (or push out) for three seconds, hold for a second, and then lower the

weight to a count of three seconds. Always maintain control; never drop or crash your weights.
• Don't forget to stretch.

## Flexibility Training

Stretching helps to enhance the flexibility of our muscles. This can help prevent injury, maintain range of motion, improve posture, promote relaxation, and make other kinds of exercise easier. We tend to lose our flexibility as we age, but if we keep stretching we can improve.

In general, you should do your stretching *after* your aerobic and strength training exercises so that your muscles are already warmed up. Stretching is easy to do at home. Aim to perform each exercise three to five times, and try to hold the stretch for ten to thirty seconds. Do not stretch to the point of pain. To try to stretch a muscle further, relax a minute, take a deep breath, and then stretch again as you breathe out. Never bounce, and never lock your joints. *Remember, don't hang your head upside down.* This can raise IOP.

Yoga is a form of exercise that helps you stretch while enhancing the mind–body connection. It is fine for patients with glaucoma to practice yoga as long as they avoid inverted (upside-down) positions. I will talk more about yoga for stress reduction later in this chapter.

## Balance/Stability Training

As we get older, our risk of falling increases. Falling can lead to many types of injuries, including broken hips. Keeping your balance can help prevent this type of dangerous fall.

Strength training for your lower body can help enhance your balance. You can also practice standing first on one leg, then the other, several times each day—without holding on. See if you can do it while your eyes are closed.

Any standing strength exercise can become a balance exercise if you perform it without holding on to the table or chair in front of you, or if you hold on with only one hand or finger. Better yet, close your eyes *and* try to avoid holding on.

## A Few Words of Caution

- In addition to checking with your ophthalmologist regarding your glaucoma, be sure to consult your general health care practitioner (internist) before you begin an exercise program—especially if you suffer from a chronic ailment such as cardiovascular disease, congestive heart failure, or diabetes; if you are obese; or if you smoke.
- If you have diabetes and take oral medication or insulin, your doctor will need to adjust your dose so your blood sugar does not fall too low during and after exercise.
- If you feel faint or dizzy, while you are exercising, stop immediately and seek medical help.
- Remember that upside-down yoga positions, scuba diving, and bungee jumping should be avoided, because they can raise IOP.

## Staying Hydrated

Staying hydrated is important for everyone who exercises. This means you should drink water before, during, and after your workout. If you exercise when you are even mildly dehydrated, you won't have your normal levels of endurance or strength, and you may get dizzy. Don't wait until you become thirsty. Thirst is a sign that you are already dehydrated.

Although patients with glaucoma need water as much as anyone does, it is very important not to drink large quantities of fluids too quickly. Doing so can cause a temporary rise in IOP. Instead, concentrate on drinking a few ounces at a time, every fifteen minutes or so, throughout your entire workout period.

## EXERCISE AND PIGMENTARY GLAUCOMA

As you recall, in pigment dispersion syndrome and pigmentary glaucoma, pigment from the iris is easily liberated and can reduce the flow of aqueous through the trabecular meshwork (drain). This can lead to elevated IOP. When patients with pigmentary dispersion syndrome or pigmentary glaucoma jog—or participate in other, similarly jarring sports—they may develop an exercise-induced release of pigment from the iris and possibly an associated spike in IOP. This does *not* necessarily mean that these patients must avoid these activities. But they do need to check with their ophthalmologist, who may want to evaluate them both before and after an exercise session (especially a session that includes jarring- and bouncing-type exercises). If exercise-induced pigment dispersion with IOP elevation occurs, the doctor might initiate therapy with pilocarpine (which decreases the incidence of pigment dispersion) or an alternative medication to help blunt any associated spikes in IOP.

## OTHER ALTERNATIVE THERAPIES

In an attempt to take control of their own health and well-being, many Americans have chosen to explore alternative therapies such as acupuncture, meditation, yoga, and biofeedback.

There is no compelling clinical evidence that any of these therapies is useful in the treatment of glaucoma. However, *with the exception of marijuana*, as long as patients continue to take their medications as prescribed, most of these practices are harmless. In fact, they may enhance relaxation and encourage optimism. A positive outlook can never hurt. And it has been suggested that elevated stress levels may be associated with elevated IOP.

Before discussing acceptable alternative therapies, I want to emphasize and review the alternative treatment that should be avoided.

### What Not to Do: Marijuana

Marijuana and its derivatives have been documented to lower IOP temporarily when administered orally, intravenously, or by smoking. This drug's short duration of action makes it a highly impractical treatment for twenty-four-hour control of IOP. More important, we also know that marijuana and its derivatives lower IOP by reducing the blood flow to the ciliary body, thus reducing the amount of aqueous produced. Doctors now believe that glaucoma damage can occur when there is reduced blood flow to the eye and its fragile optic nerve. The harmful effects associated with reduced blood flow to the eye *completely negate* any beneficial effect of temporarily lowering the IOP. Marijuana can also cause significant side effects, including increased heart rate, impaired memory and concentration, impaired motor coordination, and systemic hypotension (low blood pressure). *In short, the bad effects outweigh the good—by far!*

Based on the current body of scientific knowledge, marijuana (and its derivatives) should *not* be considered an alternative to traditional glaucoma therapies. Despite this fact, some patient groups are fighting to have marijuana and/or its derivatives legalized for the treatment of glaucoma.

### Acupuncture: An Acceptable Therapy

Acupuncture is a form of ancient Chinese medicine based on the theory that an invisible life force called ch'i or qi (pronounced *chee*) flows through the body along invisible, interconnected channels called meridians. Acupuncturists access this energy by using needles to stimulate any of approximately 365 acupuncture points along these meridians. The various organs of the body correspond to various points along the meridians. Supposedly, acupuncture unblocks the flow of qi through the meridians, eventually restoring balance to the corresponding part of the body. This is a very simple explanation for a form of healing that has been practiced in China for more than five thousand years.

Although there are a few anecdotal reports of acupuncture enhancing visual acuity and lowering IOP, its use as a treatment for glaucoma has not been well studied. Acupuncture should be considered only as an adjunct to traditional treatment modalities such as eyedrops, laser, and surgery.

### Another Good Therapy: Stress Reduction

*To date, doctors do not fully understand all the effects of stress on health.* As I mentioned earlier, stress *may* be associated with elevated IOP. If stress can raise IOP, it should follow that reducing stress through biofeedback or meditation would reduce IOP. However, this effect has not been documented in clinical studies. Nonetheless, stress reduction techniques can play a valuable role in helping patients deal with the daily strain of coping with glaucoma.

There are a number of methods for dealing with stress.

- *Biofeedback:* When you practice biofeedback, you learn to control some of your physiological processes such as heart rate, muscle tension, and blood pressure through various mental exercises and techniques. To learn how to do this, your body needs to be hooked up to monitoring equipment. The type of required monitoring equipment depends on the physiological process being evaluated. A biofeedback specialist helps you use the monitors to visualize the effects of your mental activity on the bodily function being evaluated. Through specific thought processes, you learn to actually alter your heart rate, blood pressure, and breathing. Eventually, you should be able to use mental imagery and thought processes to control those processes without needing monitors.

- *Meditation* provides a short escape from the demands of daily life. There are many different forms of meditation, but most involve sitting quietly, focusing the mind, and freeing it from thoughts of the everyday world—even for just a brief time. Meditation has been scientifically proven to reduce levels of stress hormones, lower blood pressure, reduce heart rate, and provide a host of other health benefits.

Finding the time to meditate may be a significant hurdle, especially in today's hectic, fast-paced world. Many believe that *making the time* is worthwhile. Being creative about finding the time is key. (An exceptionally creative friend of mine chooses to meditate while in the backseat of a New York City taxicab as it maneuvers its way—often slowly—to her next workday meeting!)

- *Yoga* involves a series of movements and body positions. Most types of yoga include meditation and breathing exercises. There is also an element of spirituality in many forms of yoga. Although the specific goals of yoga vary according to the type you practice, most forms strengthen and stretch the muscles, improve posture, and allow relaxation.

The long-term effects of repeatedly assuming a position in which the body is inverted (head-down), as is sometimes the case in yoga, may have the potential to increase IOP. Therefore, people with glaucoma should be careful about performing exercises such as headstands and shoulder stands. If you have glaucoma and practice yoga, let your eye doctor know if those movements are part of your regular routine. Your doctor may want to alter your yoga routine accordingly.

# Part III

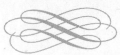

# RECENT ADVANCES

## Chapter 12

# Cutting-Edge Research That Has Revolutionized Treatment

Some recent breakthroughs in the treatment of glaucoma have resulted not from the development of new medications, novel surgical techniques, or exotic therapeutic alternatives, but as a result of meticulously designed, controlled clinical trials. These studies examined how, why, and when doctors treat both glaucoma patients and patients who are at high risk for developing glaucoma. Doctors were searching for scientific evidence to guide them with regard to whom to treat, when to treat, and how aggressively to treat. The results of these studies have truly revolutionized doctors' approaches to treating ocular hypertension (OHT) and glaucoma. Now, instead of basing treatment choices primarily on case reports or individual experience, decisions about glaucoma therapy can be based on the results of these rigorous studies. Glaucoma doctors now rely heavily on what is termed evidence-based medicine in their decision-making process.

The following studies examined four different populations: individuals with elevated intraocular pressure (IOP) that had *not* been diagnosed with glaucoma (OHT); individuals with newly detected open-angle glaucoma; individuals with advanced glaucoma; and individuals with normal-tension glaucoma (NTG).

## THE OCULAR HYPERTENSION TREATMENT STUDY (OHTS)

This groundbreaking, landmark study evaluated the crucial question: Does early treatment of IOP in people with ocular hypertension delay or prevent the onset of optic nerve damage?

The Ocular Hypertension Treatment Study evaluated 1,636 people, ages forty through eighty, who had elevated IOP without signs of glaucoma. These individuals were randomized into two groups. Members of one group took eyedrops to lower IOP (the treatment group); the other group took no medication (the observation group). In the treatment group, the goal was to reduce IOP by 20 percent or more, or to lower IOP to 24 mm Hg or less.

Researchers found that lowering the IOP in these OHT patients reduced the rate of progression to glaucoma in a statistically significant way—by more than 50 percent, as compared to the OHT patients who were not treated. Study results showed that only 4.4 percent of OHT study participants who received treatment developed glaucoma within five years. In comparison, 9.5 percent of individuals who were not medicated (observation group) went on to develop glaucoma within five years. Statistically, those OHT individuals without treatment developed glaucoma *at more than twice the rate* of the treated group. Certain ocular characteristics were also associated with a higher risk of glaucoma development. As a result of this study, physicians now consider initiating therapy for ocular hypertension patients who are at moderate or high risk of developing open-angle glaucoma *before they actually develop the disease.* Treatment to lower IOP is now initiated earlier in these individuals than before this study. Also, the OHTS study data have provided new insight into those OHT patients who are at greatest risk of progression to glaucoma. In fact, OHTS was really the first well-conceived attempt to introduce the concept of risk assessment and risk analysis for glaucoma.

The OHTS trial confirms the importance of IOP control in the treatment and pathogenesis of glaucoma. It is important to remember, however, that the results of OHTS *do not imply* that all people with elevated IOP need to be treated! OHTS reaffirms the concept that to accurately assess a patient's risk for glaucoma, physicians should evaluate the cup-to-disc ratio, which is a significant risk factor. OHTS also encourages doctors to consider measuring central corneal thickness (CCT) in determining glaucoma risk. Both cup-to-disc ratio and CCT were found to be important risk factors and powerful predictors of progression to open-angle glaucoma in this study of ocular hypertensives. (Patients with larger cup-to-disc ratios and those with thin CCTs had greater risk.) Using information such as age, cup-to-disc ratio, and IOP, in combination with CCT, allows even more valuable risk analysis.

Many unanswered questions remain, however, and new questions have arisen from the OHTS trial. Some glaucoma specialists have commented on the fact that race did not appear as a significant risk factor for glaucoma in this study. Surprisingly, other factors previously indicated as risk factors for the development of glaucoma—including gender, cardiovascular status, family history, diabetes, and hypertension—were not found to be significant in this study. This result may be a product of how the study was designed.

234 What Your Doctor May Not Tell You About Glaucoma

Clearly, more studies of OHT patients are required. Fortunately, the patients in the OHTS trial are still being followed, and new information will emerge as additional years of data are analyzed and published in the glaucoma peer-reviewed journals (OHTS 2).

## EARLY MANIFEST GLAUCOMA TRIAL (EMGT)

The Early Manifest Glaucoma Trial was the first well-conceived, well-controlled study to answer the questions: Do patients with glaucoma do better when treated to lower the IOP than glaucoma patients who are not treated? Does treating the glaucoma by lowering IOP really slow the progression of the disease?

Prior to this study, doctors already believed that lowering IOP was beneficial, but there were no well-designed clinical trials to document those beliefs. For this reason, the EMGT became a landmark study: It finally documented that treatment of glaucoma does make a difference, and can indeed alter visual field progression and optic nerve deterioration.

The EMGT was a prospective, multicenter trial performed in Sweden. The study followed 255 patients, ages fifty-five through eighty, with newly diagnosed early-stage glaucoma in at least one eye. Subjects were randomized into two groups. One group of patients (129 individuals) received treatment; the other patients (126 individuals) were observed. The maximum IOP allowed in study patients was 32 mm Hg. This was felt to be the highest level of IOP that could possibly be safe for a glaucoma patient who was randomized to a nontreatment group. Researchers believed that nontreatment of an IOP greater than 32 mm Hg could prove too dangerous for the patient.

To participate in the EMGT study, patients needed to have visual field defects consistent with glaucoma. However, it was required that their visual fields showed early damage only, rather than advanced damage. Entry into the nontreatment group would prove too risky for patients in whom the visual field showed very significant, advanced-stage glaucomatous damage.

The medical intervention provided to the study group receiving treatment was a regimen that was considered optimal and the safest at the time (early 1990s): Betoptic (betaxalol) and argon laser trabeculoplasty (ALT). No specific target IOP was set.

Researchers evaluated the progression of glaucoma in study subjects by monitoring visual field test results and observing changes in the optic nerve head (disc). Researchers used very sensitive criteria to determine visual field progression. Patients were observed over a six-year period.

At the end of the six-year study period, researchers determined that there was a difference between the two groups. The rate of progression of glaucoma was 62 percent in the observation group, and only 45 percent in the treatment group—a statistically significant difference.

It should be noted that the progression rates for glaucoma seen in this study are higher than other studies have found. This can probably be explained by the fact that *progression* was defined very sensitively, so that any subtle change in the visual field was considered to demonstrate progression. In addition, on average, the treatment (betaxalol plus ALT) achieved only a 25 percent reduction in IOP. This was *not* a maximal reduction of IOP chosen to ensure optimal stability of the optic nerve and visual field. In other words, medication and laser were given and the IOP responded, but no additional medications or treatments were added to further lower the IOP to bring it to a specific target level. (For example, in treating glaucoma—depending on the specifics of the individual patient—most glaucoma doctors recommend a 20 to 40 percent reduction in IOP. A 25 percent IOP reduction—as was achieved, on average, in this study—is *not* considered aggressive management of glaucoma.)

Analysis of the EMGT data revealed another, significant statistic that is often quoted by doctors today: During follow-up, *there is a 10 percent reduction in risk of glaucoma progression for each additional 1 mm Hg IOP reduction.* Analysts reached this conclusion by making a dose–response curve and plotting the IOP reductions obtained against rate of disease progression. (Interestingly, the OHTS results included a similar statistic. IOP is also a risk factor for *developing* glaucoma among the studied OHT patients. For each additional 1 mm Hg IOP, the risk of developing glaucoma was increased by about 10 percent.)

## The Impact of EMGT

This landmark study has affected the way doctors think about glaucoma treatment. The EMGT was successful in answering the question researchers had been asking for years: Is there a clinical benefit to glaucoma treatment? The answer was clearly yes: *Treatment (lowering IOP) helps reduce the progression of glaucoma.* The results were consistent with those of other studies in that the more IOP could be reduced, the greater the reduction in patient risk of glaucoma progression.

How has this study affected the way doctors treat glaucoma? The EMGT gave doctors a better understanding of just how beneficial IOP reduction could be to glaucoma patients, regardless of such individual variables as cup-to-disc ratio, significance of visual field defect, initial IOP level, and so on. Furthermore, doctors contemplate and debate EMGT's interesting statistic regarding the importance of a 1 mm Hg lowering of IOP. This statistic is truly food for thought and will hopefully lead to further research in the near future.

# ADVANCED GLAUCOMA INTERVENTION STUDY (AGIS)

The purpose of the Advanced Glaucoma Intervention Study was to evaluate the outcomes of different sequences of surgical interventions in individuals with advanced glaucoma in whom medical therapy had failed to provide adequate treatment.

AGIS was a randomized, controlled clinical trial of 591 patients with advanced glaucoma (789 eyes), ages thirty-five through eighty, with seven years of follow-up. Patients were randomized into two groups. The first underwent argon laser trabeculoplasty (ALT) and then trabeculectomy if ALT failed, followed by another trabeculectomy if the first failed. The second group underwent trabeculectomy followed by ALT if the trabeculectomy failed, followed by a second trabeculectomy if the ALT failed.

After seven years, AGIS results showed that blacks and whites responded to these surgical treatment sequences in different ways. The vision in black patients was better preserved by the treatment sequence that began with ALT. In white patients, vision was better preserved with laser surgery during the first four years of the study. Thereafter, though, the reverse was true. Seven years after the initial treatment, white patients who began treatment with trabeculectomy had less vision loss.

Based on the results of the AGIS study, some doctors recommend that black patients with advanced glaucoma undergo ALT as their initial surgical treatment rather than trabeculectomy. However, white patients with advanced glaucoma and no life-threatening health problems would more often be recommended to initiate surgical treatment with trabeculectomy. (It should be noted that no Mitomycin-C was used in this study.)

AGIS study results have shown that both whites and blacks have a good response to argon laser trabeculoplasty, suggesting that ALT is a reasonable first option for either group. In addition, AGIS results indicate that trabeculectomy *without* Mitomycin-C (MMC) works less well in blacks, but better results may be seen in blacks when MMC is used.

AGIS gave doctors insight into the question of whether an IOP reduction of as little as 1, 2, or 3 mm Hg makes a real difference in terms of glaucoma progression. AGIS has helped doctors determine how low the IOP must go in order to avoid glaucoma progression. The advanced glaucoma patients in AGIS were followed over eight to nine years. They were analyzed by group according to average IOP: average IOP less than 14 mm Hg; average IOP of 14 to 17 mm Hg; average IOP of 18 mm Hg and above. Over time, the group that achieved and maintained the lowest IOP (less than 14 mm Hg) levels had the least risk of glaucoma progression. In fact, the mean visual field loss was *three times greater* in patients with IOP between 14 and 17.5 mm Hg as compared to patients with IOP less than 14 mm Hg! Therefore, there is clearly a difference between having an IOP of less than 14 mm Hg and one of 18 mm Hg. At three to four years, the differences among the groups were not as extreme. But as the years went on, the differences became increasingly significant.

AGIS has helped doctors consider glaucoma treatment as a long-term proposition. In the treatment of patients with advanced glaucoma, it is important to lower IOP, closely monitor the patient to be sure this lowered IOP is maintained, and to understand that a significant benefit will be reaped eight to ten years down the road: Patients will have significantly less glaucoma progression.

Another interesting finding from the AGIS study is the importance of diurnal IOP control. Not only is the mean IOP important, but the stability of IOP levels was also found to be of significance. The group with the least visual field progression included those patients whose IOP was consistently (at all visits) under 18 mm Hg. A consistently low IOP reduces vision loss—it stabilizes the visual field. AGIS demonstrated the importance of maintaining a consistently low IOP over time. After surgery to reduce IOP, patients whose IOP levels were always below 18 mm Hg over the six-year follow-up period had visual field progression close to zero. In this group with minimal glaucoma progression, the mean IOP was 12.3 mm Hg. The progression rate for patients for whom IOP was less than 18 mm Hg during 75 to 100 percent of visits was significantly higher. *Tight diurnal IOP control, not just a low average (mean) IOP, is significant.*

Today doctors have become much more aggressive in terms of IOP-lowering efforts. Since patients live longer, doctors must consider lifelong risk—not just stability in the short term. So if doctors can lower (and consistently sustain) the IOP even just 1, 2, or 3 additional mm Hg, this may provide additional long-term stability to glaucoma patients. Doctors and patients have much more information to consider when deciding whether it is worth it to put up with some medication-related side effects in order to lower IOP by a few additional mm Hg. Clearly, AGIS data support the concept that an IOP of less than 14 mm Hg helps stabilize the visual field and reduce glaucoma progression. But keep in mind that when doctors think of glaucoma management for the long term and going for the lowest safe IOP, they still must weigh the three key factors in choosing treatments: efficacy, safety, and tolerability. All things being equal, though, choosing a regimen that lowers IOP to the greatest possible extent (without being too low or hypotonous) is probably going to be of greatest long-term benefit to the patient with glaucoma.

## THE COLLABERATIVE INITIAL GLAUCOMA TREATMENT STUDY (CIGTS)

This study's objective was to determine if patients newly diagnosed with primary open-angle glaucoma (POAG) are better treated initially with medication or filtration surgery. CIGTS followed these newly diagnosed patients for five years. There were 307 patients in the medication group and 300 in the surgery group.

The results of CIGTS showed that initial treatment with either medications or trabeculectomy was effective in lowering IOP over a five-year follow-up period. More important, both initial medical treatment and initial surgery were effective in stabilizing the visual fields of these POAG patients. During the first three years of this study, visual field loss was greater in the surgery group than in the medication group. By years four and five, these differences in visual field loss disappeared.

CIGTS is an important study. It confirmed that no matter how the IOP was significantly lowered (whether by medications or filtering surgery) in patients with newly diagnosed POAG, doctors can stabilize the visual field and halt glaucoma progression. Unfortunately, CIGTS included only a five-year follow-up. Most glaucoma doctors agree that five years of follow-up is not adequate for making conclusions about treatments for this chronic disease.

## COLLABORATIVE NORMAL-TENSION GLAUCOMA GROUP (CNTG)

The Collaborative Normal-Tension Glaucoma Group (CNTG) revealed that lowering the IOP in normal-tension glaucoma patients (with glaucoma damage that occurs at normal IOP levels) was beneficial in preserving visual field. Lowered IOP in NTG patients slows or halts vision loss (loss of visual field).

In this study, one eye of NTG patients was randomized to IOP-lowering treatment or to no treatment. Eyes that maintained a 30 percent reduction in IOP showed significantly less progression of optic disc cupping and/or visual field changes. In the untreated group, the glaucoma progression rate was 35 percent versus only 12 percent in the treated group.

The CNTG study gave doctors clear evidence that lowering the IOP by 30 percent is beneficial in protecting the visual field—even for glaucoma patients who are known to develop glaucomatous damage at "normal" levels of IOP.

Overall, these landmark studies confirmed the benefit of lowering IOP in an effort to reduce the risk of progressive visual field loss and optic nerve damage. These trials provided doctors with *real evidence* that lowering IOP was beneficial for a wide range of individuals—from the person with elevated IOP with no glaucoma damage (ocular hypertension) to the one with advanced glaucomatous visual field loss.

Using this evidence-based medicine, many doctors are concluding that IOP-lowering efforts should be initiated *earlier* and *more aggressively.* Hopefully, additional well-designed research studies like these will provide doctors with even more evidence to guide their decisions regarding the best ways to manage glaucoma and OHT. Future well-designed clinical trials will help doctors develop better risk profiles for patients with glaucoma and OHT. By identifying risk factors, doctors will be better able to determine an individual's risk of glaucoma progression and better determine an optimal, individualized treatment regimen to preserve vision and visual function throughout the individual's lifetime.

*Chapter 13*

# Innovations in Diagnostic Testing and Monitoring

The three most important diagnostic clues for glaucoma are:

1. Damage to the optic nerve, seen as increased cupping of the optic nerve head and/or other changes in the disc, such as disc hemorrhages or notching.
2. Visual field loss that usually—but not always—starts peripherally.
3. Intraocular pressure (IOP) that is usually—but not always—elevated.

However, since *glaucoma can exist without elevated IOP* and *elevated IOP can exist without glaucoma*, the status of the optic nerve and visual field must be accurately assessed to diagnose glaucoma and monitor its progress. New technologies now allow doctors to more precisely evaluate the health of the optic nerve and more accurately measure the extent of vision loss (loss of visual field).

It is important to remember that the standard eye checkup for glaucoma involves direct examination of the optic nerve head (disc). This is usually accomplished using a direct oph-thalmoscope or a magnifying lens with the slit lamp. Sketches of the optic disc by the doctor or photographs (sometimes stereoscopic) document the disc's appearance. Today, however, sophisticated imaging devices help doctors assess the optic nerve and document its health in ways that far exceed the methods used in the standard eye checkup. In addition, new forms of visual field tests have been and are being developed that facilitate earlier diagnosis of glaucoma, shorten testing time, improve test precision, and make visual field testing more useful and reliable in patients with blurred vision.

*Unfortunately, not all doctors who care for glaucoma patients have these latest devices to image the optic nerve head and assess the visual field more precisely. These instruments, being expensive, are most likely to be found in the offices of glaucoma specialists and the medical teaching institutions.*

## VISUAL FIELD TESTING (PERIMETRY)

Visual field testing has advanced greatly in recent years. Some experts estimate that glaucoma damage can be detected as much as five years earlier using newer techniques than with the standard white-on-white (white stimuli on a white background) visual field used in Humphrey perimetry, the current standard among glaucoma doctors. (See discussion of visual fields in chapter 10.) Earlier diagnosis means earlier treatment, and earlier treatment can prevent the optic nerve from developing early glaucoma damage, thus preserving sight. The newer tests also allow doctors to detect and monitor visual field changes more easily.

The two new kinds of visual field testing are called short wavelength automated perimetry (SWAP) and frequency doubling technology perimetry (FDT). These new technologies work by testing different groups or types of retinal ganglion cells (the cells that are destroyed in glaucoma). The first group of ganglion cells is very responsive to slow changes and fine details. The second group is sensitive to the color blue. A third group is responsive to rapid changes in frequency. These new tests are especially important in confirming whether a person truly has a visual field abnormality. They also help doctors determine whether subsequent visual field tests show real changes or just variability among tests. The use of SWAP and FDT, in combination with standard white-on-white perimetry, is likely to become the norm in the near future.

### Short Wavelength Automated Perimetry (SWAP)

SWAP is performed on the Humphrey visual field machine (perimeter) and is the so-called blue-on-yellow test. This test shows the patient blue stimuli (dots of light) on a yellow background. For a patient to detect these blue dots on a yellow background, a specific ganglion cell must function. It is these specific ganglion cells that are being tested in SWAP.

*The SWAP test is more sensitive in early glaucoma than late and can detect visual field loss before it would be detected with a standard white-on-white test.* However, there are some disadvantages to the SWAP test. For instance, there is great variability among tests. The testing time for SWAP is usually greater than standard white-on-white perimetry. Cataracts reduce its accuracy. Furthermore, patients with advanced visual field damage may not be able to detect many of the blue-on-yellow stimuli (dots), and this test may not be very helpful for them.

*SWAP is best for young patients with no cataracts who are being evaluated for possible early glaucoma.* It is less helpful when trying to detect disease progression in patients already diagnosed with glaucoma.

A faster version of SWAP is being developed. This will be highly beneficial in helping SWAP to gain wide acceptance by patients and doctors.

### Frequency Doubling Technology (FDT)

Frequency doubling technology (FDT) measures a form of contrast sensitivity. There are fewer points of vision tested than in standard perimetry. FDT tests the central twenty to thirty degrees of vision. It is a rapid test that usually takes less than five minutes. Unlike white-on-white perimetry, patients do *not* have to be in a dimly lit room for the FDT. *This test is useful in patients who have blurred vision or cataracts* since results are not affected by an inability to focus.

An advantage of the FDT is that it is very effective at early detection and is extremely useful as a screening tool. In fact, FDT is currently most often used in a screening-type setting when many people are being tested and screened for glaucoma. The FDT perimeter is very portable and relatively inexpensive. A disadvantage of the FDT perimeter test is that it tests only a small number of locations in the patient's field of vision. A new version is currently being developed that tests more spots and will be more useful.

## OTHER NEW VISUAL TESTING DEVICES

### High Pass Resolution Perimetry (HRP)

HRP was developed in Sweden and is not readily available in the United States. This test uses a video monitor to present images of rings of various sizes to a patient. The rings consist of a very light central area surrounded by a darker ring.

HRP has provided results that are similar to standard perimetry. HRP is reported to have a better consistency among test results than standard white-on-white perimetry, especially in patients who have significant visual field loss as a result of glaucoma. Some studies have concluded that HRP can detect progression of visual field in glaucoma *one to two years earlier* than conventional white-on-white perimetry. In addition, patients find HRP very user-friendly because it is faster, interactive, and gives the patient feedback during the test. Significant disadvantages of the HRP, however, include a lack of standardization in equipment and limited technical support.

### Swedish Interactive Thresholding Algorithm (SITA)

SITA was developed by Zeiss Humphrey and is considered by many glaucoma specialists to be the current gold standard of visual field testing. The advantage of this test is that the doctor is able to obtain reliable and accurate information in a brief period of time—five to ten minutes. By keeping the test time brief, patients are more able to concentrate and sit still during the visual field test, but doctors still get the data they need to find the threshold of the visual field accurately. Finding the threshold involves answering the question: How bright must the stimulus be for the patient to just be able to detect it? In my own experience, the SITA has made fewer patients dread the visual field test. Suprisingly, some patients enjoy it.

*Glaucoma doctors usually consider visual field testing to be one of the most important—if not* the *most important—test performed on patients with glaucoma or suspicion of glaucoma.* The visual field test is an important test of visual functioning and can also reveal medical problems other than glaucoma, such as neurological problems related to sight—stroke, brain tumors, inflammation of the optic nerve, and more. The SITA test facilitates this because instead of using one standard test, it customizes the test to the individual based on that individual patient's responses, thresholds, and pacing requirements.

SITA comes in two forms: SITA standard and SITA fast. As compared to standard visual field testing on the Humphrey machine, SITA standard reduces the testing time by 50 percent and SITA fast reduces the testing time by 70 percent. Among the SITA tests, there are two forms of each of the above two: 24-2 (said *24 dash 2*) and 30-2 (*30 dash 2*). The 24-2 tests the central twenty-four degrees of visual field. The 30-2 tests the central thirty degrees of visual field. In addition to these, there is also a 10-2 test of the central ten degrees of field and a 60-4 test of the central sixty degrees of field. These are less commonly used, but are appropriate in certain patients. Many glaucoma specialists now consider their standard visual field test to be the SITA standard 24-2.

### The Future of Visual Field Testing

Doctors expect future visual field tests to become more rapid and more customized to the individual patient. SWAP and FDT will be employed more often to provide doctors with an improved ability to detect the earliest of visual field defects and to better compare visual field tests over time. With these tests, earlier detection of glaucoma and better monitoring of glaucoma will be a reality.

## ADDITIONAL DIAGNOSTIC TESTS

### Visual Evoked Response (VER) or Visual Evoked Potential (VEP)

The VER is the electrical response generated by the brain (specifically, the occipital visual cortex) when the retina is stimulated with light. In this test, light is presented to the retina as either flashes or patterns (checkerboards). When light flashes are used, this is called flash VER. When light patterns are presented, this is called pattern VER.

Among the different VERs, researchers believe that the pattern VER is the most helpful in evaluating a patient's visual pathway. It is very sensitive, and is an objective way to evaluate abnormalities of the optic nerve and anterior visual pathway—particularly in glaucoma.

## The Multifocal ERG (Electroretinogram)

Visual field tests provide an excellent way to evaluate optic nerve function, but visual fields are very subjective. Their quality depends on how alert and attentive the patient is during the test. When the patient performing the visual field test is tired, distracted, or does not fully understand the test, the results are not ideal.

Today researchers continue to look for more objective ways to test for optic nerve damage related to glaucoma. An objective test, by definition, is not dependent on variables such as fatigue, distraction, or poor comprehension.

The ERG is an objective test of retinal function. It involves stimulating a person's retina in a very specific way, with a very specific target. The retina's response to the stimulus is recorded with an electrode on the eye.

The most commonly used ERG is the full-field ERG. It tests the response of the retina to very large stimuli and is a poor test for glaucoma-related damage. This standard ERG measures a nonspecific mass response of the retina and is unable to look for localized changes in the retina. Another form of the ERG is called the pattern ERG. This test examines the retinal ganglion cells, but it has been found to have a low specificity for glaucoma changes. Pattern ERG is not useful in glaucoma evaluation and management.

The most promising form of ERG is the multifocal ERG (mERG). This is an exciting new tool in the evaluation of glaucoma. Unlike the standard ERG, mERG is able to look at localized retinal responses. The test is objective and does not depend upon subjective patient variables such as fatigue and concentration.

During the mERG, over one hundred areas of the retina are stimulated at the exact same time. A contact lens electrode on the eye measures the retinal responses. The result is a map of the retina that shows the responsiveness in each of the different areas tested. The mERG is able to detect changes in patients who are suspected of having glaucoma but who do *not* have an abnormal visual field.

At present, multifocal ERG testing is still experimental. In the future, however, this test may give doctors an objective way to detect early, glaucoma-related abnormalities of the retinal ganglion cells long before the visual field would be affected. For this reason, mERG holds great promise in the evaluation and management of glaucoma patients.

## IMAGING THE INTERIOR OF THE EYE

Years ago, when a doctor evaluated a glaucoma patient, he or she could only rely upon hand-drawn sketches of the optic nerve head to record its appearance and health status and document such factors as whether or not the disc was cupped, the cup-to-disc ratio, disc hemorrhages, and more. As technology advanced, doctors were able to take stereoscopic disc photographs that recorded the appearance of the optic nerve head in greater detail and with enhanced reliably. But today, doctors can use computerized imaging devices to identify, document, and follow even the most subtle changes in the optic nerve head.

Determining the cup-to-disc ratio and evaluating the

amount of cupping are important, but modern glaucoma doctors need and want to look for much more. We also want to assess the integrity of the neural rim, the amount of peripapillary (next-to-the-disc) atrophy, and defects in the retinal nerve fiber layer (RNFL).

Research has shown that damage to the RNFL occurs before visual field changes are seen in early glaucoma, and today's newest technologies provide the objectivity and accuracy to meaningfully image the retinal nerve fiber layer. These new technologies include confocal scanning laser ophthalmoscopy (CSLO), scanning laser polarimetry (SLP), and optical coherence tomography (OCT).

### Confocal Scanning Laser Ophthalmoscopy (CSLO)

This technology is being used in Heidelberg Retinal Tomography (HRT) (figure 32). The Heidelberg provides three-dimensional (3-D) analysis of the optic nerve head topography. In this procedure, a low-energy laser light scans the retina in two directions. The images that are produced contain approximately 150,000 pixels and are full of information.

Once the image is generated, a technician manually outlines the margin of the optic disc. Analysis of this data is then performed by the software within the HRT. The neural rim and the optic cup are clearly delineated. The software then calculates the depth of the optic cup, the contours of the disc, and other parameters that help doctors evaluate the optic nerve head. These include disc area, rim area, cup area, cup and rim volumes, cup-to-disc ratios, horizontal and vertical cup-to-disc ratios, retinal nerve fiber layer thickness, and more. Researchers have found that the data provided by the HRT are highly reproducible.

One challenge that researchers are tackling is the issue of change analysis. Researchers are attempting to develop a

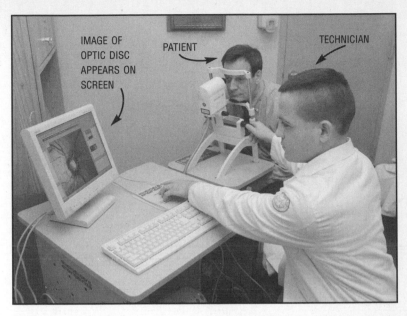

**Figure 32.** Heidelberg retinal tomography (HRT): The technician is adjusting the image of the patient's optic disc on the screen.

method by which Heidelberg HRT images that have been performed over time on a single patient can be analyzed to determine whether there have been changes. The difficulty is that tests can show variability from one to another without being truly different.

HRT is an excellent device in the analysis of the optic nerve head, and it does not require the patient's pupils to be dilated. It does, however, have certain limitations. HRT requires the operator or technician to correctly identify the margins of the disc. If not done properly, this can lead to errors. In addition, HRT technology cannot identify certain specific changes in the optic nerve head that are often seen with progression. These changes include disc pallor, disc hemorrhage, and the shifting of blood vessels to one side (the nasal side) of the disc.

## Scanning Laser Polarimetry (SLP)

SLP allows doctors to image the optic nerve head (without dilating the pupil) and evaluate the retinal nerve fiber layer that lies adjacent to the optic nerve head (the peripapillary RNFL). In SLP technology, a polarized diode laser light (780 nanometers) is used to scan the retina. The instrument using SLP technology is called the GDx.

In this technology, at least three images are required. Color maps of the optic nerve head and the retinal nerve fiber layers adjacent to the disc (peripapillary) are made. The computer analyzes each quadrant of the optic nerve head. SLP identifies the thickest and thinnest parts of the RNFL.

This technology has its limitations. The SLP depends upon measuring the amount of retardance or delay of polarized light as it passes through the tissues of the eye (primarily the retina) for its determinations, yet the cornea has polarization that can significantly affect these measurements. Researchers have shown that recently made corrections for error related to the cornea in the newest version of the GDx (GDxVCC) have increased this technology's ability to detect early to moderate glaucoma.

## Optical Coherence Tomography (OCT)

OCT produces cross-sectional images of the retina. This technology allows accurate measurements of the peripapillary (next-to-the-disc) retinal nerve fiber layer, the optic disc, and the macula (the center of the retina and the surrounding area of the retina that provide you with the sharpest central vision).

The ability of this technology to evaluate the macula is of great significance. In glaucoma, the characteristic and final common pathway is the loss of retinal ganglion cells and their axons. Research has shown that there is a substantial loss of retinal ganglion cells in the macula of monkeys with glaucoma. Thus, studying the macula is very relevant to doctors' understanding of glaucoma. In addition, recent studies have shown that changes in visual function and retinal nerve fiber layer thickness in glaucoma correlate well with macular thickness. Measurements of the retinal nerve fiber layer by OCT also correlate well with visual field defects.

The OCT imaging device is noninvasive. The device can image retinal structures with resolution up to ten to seventeen microns. OCT uses near-infrared light (850 nanometers) produced by a diode laser.

In OCT, there is circular scanning of the retinal nerve fiber layer. Approximately a hundred axial scans are used in one evaluation. The OCT software converts all of these scans into a single image. The retinal nerve fiber layer thickness is measured. The most recent version of the OCT uses 512 individual scans and has a resolution of seven to eight microns. An image has 512,000 pixels!

The patient's pupil must be dilated to obtain an image with OCT because it must be at least three millimeters in diameter (unlike the other two imaging systems, HRT and GDx).

One limitation of the technology associated with OCT is an inability to analyze the retinal nerve fiber layer thickness measurements over a period of time. Other limitations of OCT include the lack of a computer database of measurements for healthy eyes that can be used for comparative purposes. Also, OCT is unable to obtain images when there are problems such as corneal scarring, cataract, or vitreous hemorrhage.

Overall, OCT is a very promising technology that provides a sensitive and specific way of detecting and monitoring glaucoma. It has the ability to create detailed, high-resolution images of the macula and the retinal nerve fiber layer.

Currently, researchers are fine-tuning the newest version of OCT: ultra high resolution OCT (UHROCT). This instrument will revolutionize the ability of glaucoma doctors to evaluate and monitor the retinal layers. All retinal layers will be more easily visualized. UHROCT is expected to be ready for release within the next five years.

### Retinal Thickness Analyzer (RTA)

The retinal thickness analyzer (RTA) is an instrument that can image the optic disc and measure retinal thickness in the macula and peripapillary regions.

In RTA, a green laser beam made of helium and neon is projected onto the disc or retina. Light is backscattered. The reflected light is recorded by a camera. This information is then digitized. A three-by-three-millimeter area is scanned in 0.3 seconds; one scan contains sixteen cross sections. A full examination of an eye takes three to four minutes. The RTA analyzes the scans and creates 2-D and 3-D thickness maps that compare the data with data from normal individuals.

The RTA may prove very useful in the early detection of glaucoma by identifying macular and paramacular changes that *precede* visual field loss. Remember that an individual can lose up to five hundred thousand ganglion cells and still have a normal visual field. Clearly, detecting glaucoma-related damage *before* vision (visual field) loss is ideal.

Among glaucoma specialists, the most commonly used imaging systems are the HRT and GDx. OCT and RTA are used much less frequently. OCT is rapidly gaining in popularity among retinal specialists.

## ULTRASOUND BIOMICROSCOPY

Charles Pavlin and Stuart Foster were the first researchers to use very high-frequency (VHF) ultrasound in the evaluation of the anterior segment of the eye (cornea, iris, lens, anterior chamber angle, ciliary body, and so on). The transducer frequency was 50 to 80 MHz (megahertz). Their technique was termed ultrasound biomicroscopy (UBM). Prior to the development of UBM, the anterior chamber, the iris, the ciliary body, and the cornea could not be imaged well. Doctors could only use ultrasound to examine the posterior portions of the eye (retina, vitreous).

Commercially available UBM machines are most commonly seen in glaucoma practices and medical centers where they help evaluate the most challenging glaucoma cases.

In recent years, a new and exciting technique has evolved that allows ultrasound to study the fine details of the anterior segment using a very high-frequency transducer in conjunction with an immersion bath to study these anterior structures. This technique is extremely valuable in monitoring many types of glaucoma including angle-closure glaucoma, plateau iris syndrome, open-angle glaucoma, pigment dispersion glaucoma, juvenile glaucoma, and traumatic glaucoma. This technology also allows the central corneal thickness to be measured very precisely and reliably.

Currently, the technique of VHF ultrasound involves an immersion bath. The patient lies flat on a table, and a small plastic drape is positioned over the eye to hold a small amount of saline. The front surface of the eye is bathed in saline. This is completely comfortable for the patient. The ultrasound transducer is positioned into the saline but does not touch the eye. Ultrasound travels through the saline and onto the eye, creating ultrasound images of the anterior segment.

One physician and researcher who has been pivotal in developing this technology is D. Jackson Coleman, M.D., Weill Cornell Medical College, New York Presbyterian Hospital.

In the near future, Dr. Coleman and his collaborators will be releasing a new imaging system that uses very high-frequency ultrasound imaging. Using digital radio frequency data collection, the device will create three-dimensional mapping of

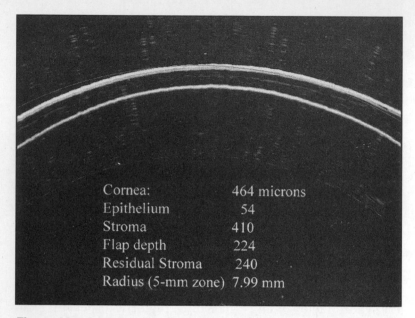

**Figure 33a.** Artemis measurements of the cornea and central corneal thickness (CCT). (Courtesy of D. Jackson Coleman, M.D.)

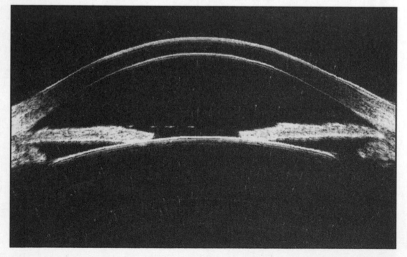

**Figure 33b.** Artemis measurements of the anterior chamber. (Courtesy of D. Jackson Coleman, M.D.)

the structures in the anterior segment of the eye. This new ultrasound technology produces a larger and more detailed scan area and allows the anterior segment to be more precisely analyzed than with current ultrasound imaging devices. It produces more accurate dimensions of the cornea, anterior chamber depth, angle, iris, ciliary body, and lens surface. The Cornell/Coleman/VHF ultrasound unit has been named Artemis 2 and will become commercially available in 2005 (figures 33a and 33b).

## MINIATURE CONTINUOUS INTRAOCULAR PRESSURE SENSOR

Continuous monitoring of IOP may be a reality in the near future. In a 2003 meeting of the Association for Research in Vision and Ophthalmology (ARVO), researchers presented the prototype of a sensor that can continuously monitor IOP via telemetry, without direct contact with the eye. The device uses a receiving pickup coil that is placed in the patient's eyeglasses. An external energy source excites the sensor's circuit. The sensor then sends out a signal that can be detected by the pickup coil. The frequency of the signal sent out by the sensor correlates with the level of IOP. With this new device, researchers will be able to better test new therapies for lowering IOP. Furthermore, twenty-four-hour monitoring of IOP in patients with glaucoma (particularly normal-tension glaucoma) and ocular hypertension will vastly improve the ability of doctors to manage these conditions.

*Chapter 14*

# Innovations in Surgery

Since surgery is a key element—and often a necessary step—in glaucoma management, the search for safer and more effective surgical techniques is crucial. Through creative thinking and innovative research, surgical advancements have been and continue to be made. Recently, for example, surgeons and researchers have developed a new surgical technique for creating a glaucoma filter *without* entering the eye. Similar degrees of innovation have led to the development of a laser trabeculoplasty that lowers intraocular pressure (IOP) without creating any scar tissue.

Let's explore the most recent and exciting innovations in surgery for glaucoma patients.

## NONPENETRATING GLAUCOMA SURGERY

As discussed in chapter 8, a standard filtering surgery (trabeculectomy) involves the removal of a small portion of the trabecular meshwork, and then covering the opening with a partial-thickness scleral flap. Fluid flows through this newly created drain or opening and out into a reservoir on the surface of the eye, called a bleb. A bleb can be described as a cyst-like elevation in the conjunctiva. To accomplish standard filtering surgery, the anterior chamber of the eye is entered.

The main thing that differentiates nonpenetrating surgery from standard filtering surgery is that the anterior chamber *is not entered*. In this new technique, the surgeon dissects through the sclera, down to the level of Descemet's membrane (the innermost layer of the cornea) but not into the anterior chamber. This dissected opening is called a sclerostomy.

Let's look at how this surgery works in more detail. Descemet's membrane is the innermost layer of the cornea. When the delicate dissection involved in this surgery is performed properly, Descemet's membrane is not penetrated. For aqueous to escape the eye, it must *percolate through this membrane* rather than through an opening in the sclera, as with a trabeculectomy.

There are clear advantages to a filtering procedure that does not require entry into the eye. By not entering the anterior chamber and by requiring that aqueous percolate through an *intact* Descemet's membrane, the risk of overfiltration, hypotony (IOP too low), or a flat anterior chamber is greatly reduced. Since the anterior chamber is never entered, the risk of cataract and infection is also reduced. These reductions in surgical risk are the key advantages of nonpenetrating glaucoma surgery.

One of the problems associated with nonpenetrating surgery is that it is a very technically challenging procedure to perform. The dissection to Descemet's membrane without entry into the anterior chamber can be difficult to master. The anterior chamber can be inadvertently entered with the slightest miscalculation, and then the surgery is *necessarily converted to a standard filtering surgery.*

Often, after nonpenetrating surgery, if the IOP is not low enough, an additional treatment that involves the YAG laser is required. The YAG laser is used to make an opening in the membrane that was so carefully dissected during surgery. By opening this membrane using laser, aqueous is able to more easily flow through the drain, thus lowering the IOP. To have a successful, nonpenetrating surgery, the dissection must be done precisely. There is very little room for error. Overall, I believe that this type of nonpenetrating surgery is best performed *only* by an experienced glaucoma surgeon.

### Deep Sclerectomy with Intrascleral Implants

In this nonpenetrating surgical procedure, popularized by Dr. Andre Mermoud, meticulous dissection (as described above) is completed. Following this dissection, an implant made of collagen is positioned within the dissected area. This implant prevents any collapse of the scleral flap. The collagen implant is made from porcine (pig) scleral collagen and dissolves within six to nine months. The space that this dissolved implant leaves behind is a space for aqueous filtration—a reservoir for aqueous to collect after leaving the anterior chamber.

### Viscocanalostomy

Viscocanalostomy is a form of nonpenetrating surgery. In this procedure, meticulous dissection of the sclera is performed. This dissection unroofs a portion of the eye's drainage system: Schlemm's canal. After Schlemm's canal is unroofed, a small tubelike instrument (cannula) is introduced into it. A very elastic substance (called viscoelastic) is injected (at high velocity) for four to six millimeters on each side of the opening into Schlemm's canal. This injection enlarges the diameter of the canal from 30 microns to 230 microns, allowing increased outflow of aqueous. Following this, a small sponge is used to place pressure on the drain and the adjacent Descemet's membrane. A small window is made in Descemet's membrane. Aqueous is able to easily pass through this window from the anterior chamber into the subscleral lake. Aqueous reaches Schlemm's canal more easily because it is able to bypass much of the resistance to outflow that is present in the inner wall or floor of Schlemm's canal. Finally, the superficial scleral flap is sutured in place.

Viscocanalostomy is generally less effective in reducing IOP than standard filtering surgery, but the risk of side effects is much lower.

### Filtering Glaucoma Surgery with Excimer Laser (Laser Trabecular Ablation, or LTA)

Laser trabecular ablation is another new nonpenetrating glaucoma filtration procedure. In this procedure, performed under topical anesthesia alone (the eye is numbed by using eyedrops and gel, not injections), a small incision is made in the conjunctiva, followed by the creation of a small scleral flap. Schlemm's canal is unroofed. Using an excimer laser, the roof and inner wall of Schlemm's canal—as well as part of the trabecular meshwork—are treated with the laser until a very small opening is seen. The scleral flap and conjunctiva are sutured closed. In this simple procedure, filtration is increased and IOP lowered, without making an opening into the anterior chamber. As a result of this surgery, aqueous flows out of the eye more easily. The complication rate is low with laser trabecular ablation. However, further evaluation of this technique is required and under way.

## Is Nonpenetrating Glaucoma Surgery a Replacement for Trabeculectomy?

In the hands of the experienced glaucoma surgeon, the rate of complications after standard filtering surgery (trabeculectomy) is very low and the success rate is high. Among U.S. glaucoma surgeons, trabeculectomy is tried and true, and able to safely lower IOP to the level needed for even patients with normal-tension glaucoma (NTG) who require very low IOPs. In contrast, nonpenetrating surgery often *does not* lower the IOP to the same degree achieved by the standard filtering surgery. For these reasons, the popularity of nonpenetrating glaucoma surgeries among U.S. glaucoma doctors has grown slowly, even though its introduction was met with great enthusiasm and excitement.

Paradoxically, although you might imagine that nonpenetrating glaucoma surgery is simple and could even be performed by someone with little experience, *the opposite is true.* The most popular forms of nonpenetrating surgery require extremely precise and exquisite dissection to be successful.

Surgeons who *are* experienced in these nonpenetrating techniques report IOP control that equals that of trabeculectomy. Other clinicians have found that the IOP control is not as good as with standard filtering surgery (trabeculectomy). However, complications such as shallow anterior chamber, hyphema (blood in the anterior chamber of the eye), choroidal detachment, and hypotony are reported to occur less often than with standard filtering surgery.

Further research and experience are required before any of these nonpenetrating techniques overcome trabeculectomy as the procedure of choice for glaucoma surgery.

# SELECTIVE LASER TRABECULOPLASTY (SLT)

SLT is an exciting new laser glaucoma therapy that may provide a real advantage over the current, standard laser therapy for many forms of open-angle glaucoma—argon laser trabeculoplasty (ALT). Unlike ALT, SLT produces no superficial scarring of the trabecular meshwork. As a result, SLT has the very exciting potential for being repeated as needed.

## ALT versus SLT

Although effective in lowering IOP, ALT does produce some harmful effects to the trabecular meshwork at a microscopic level. The argon is a thermal laser, meaning that it generates heat when applied to tissues. In ALT, heat damage occurs to the trabecular meshwork and the surrounding structural collagen fibers. Because of these structural changes (on a microscopic level) to the trabecular meshwork and the surrounding tissue, the number of times that ALT can be performed is limited—usually two or three times over a lifetime.

SLT, which uses a YAG laser, does not create thermal damage or scarring to the trabecular meshwork. Instead, SLT's laser energy is absorbed specifically by the pigmented trabecular meshwork cells *without* heat-related damage to the trabecular meshwork or the nonpigmented cells surrounding the area being treated. Endothelial membrane formation does not occur as with ALT because there is no thermal or structural damage. Theoretically, therefore, SLT can be repeated an indefinite number of times.

## SLT's Mechanism of Action

It was believed that ALT worked by causing a stretching open of the spaces within the trabecular meshwork between the laser's spots. There is no such stretching of the trabecular meshwork spaces with SLT. Instead, SLT may work at a cellular level, either through the removal of trabecular meshwork debris by macrophages or by stimulating the formation of healthy trabecular tissue.

SLT appears to increase the number of monocytes and macrophages in the trabecular meshwork. The treatment may cause a release of chemical factors that recruit macrophages to the area being treated. These macrophages clear the trabecular meshwork of debris and increase the outflow of aqueous through the drain. SLT accomplishes its pressure-lowering effect without scarring the trabecular meshwork. This is the crucial finding with SLT, and the reason that some doctors now describe SLT to patients as the "scarless trabeculoplasty."

### SLT Success Rates

Most studies show that SLT has success rates equal to those for ALT. However, unlike ALT, SLT offers the likely advantage of being able to be repeated an indefinite number of times. SLT's reported success in treating patients who have had maximal ALT treatments or failed to respond to ALT brings hope to many glaucoma patients. Studies show that SLT resulted in 70 percent of patients having an IOP reduction of at least 3 mm Hg despite an inability to control their IOP with maximal medical therapy. SLT allowed the number of glaucoma medications to be decreased significantly. The SLT procedure was found to be safe, with minimal side effects. In addition, it is exciting to see that more than 66 percent of patients who had a previous, failed ALT experienced an IOP decrease of 3 mm Hg or greater with SLT.

Recently, a number of studies have looked at the effectiveness of SLT. On average, these studies found that SLT lowered IOP by 25 percent. A British study found that SLT lowered

IOP in ocular hypertensives by 32 percent, and lowered IOP 35 percent in patients with primary open-angle glaucoma (POAG). A study done in Japan was important because the most common form of open-angle glaucoma in Asia is normal-tension glaucoma. In these patients, 68 percent saw a 20 percent reduction in IOP. Patients who had undergone a previous ALT had a success rate (20 percent reduction in IOP) of 62 percent. Other studies show that the success rate for SLT is the same for POAG patients who had previous ALT as it is for POAG patients with no previous ALT.

### The SLT Procedure

SLT is very similar to ALT. The patient is seated at the slit lamp to which the laser device is attached. The doctor uses a mirrored goniolens to examine the angle and drain. The laser device that I use is a Coherent Selecta II ophthalmic laser (YAG). The laser application is given along the trabecular meshwork in a fashion similar to ALT. The doctor looks for the release of small champagne-type bubbles from the treatment site as the laser energy is applied to the trabecular meshwork. A typical SLT treatment consists of fifty contiguous, but not overlapping, spots over 180 degrees (half the drain).

SLT is an exciting new laser treatment that is effective in lowering IOP in patients with open-angle glaucoma. Studies and clinical experience show it to be a safe alternative to ALT and a procedure that can be performed *despite failure* with ALT. Some doctors may use it as a primary treatment for patients who cannot tolerate, do not choose to, or are not compliant with glaucoma medications. In addition, the procedure has a low complication rate.

## THE EX-PRESS MINIATURE GLAUCOMA SHUNT

The Ex-PRESS shunt is a miniature, stainless-steel glaucoma shunt that was released in 2002. It measures less than three millimeters in length and four hundred microns in diameter. The shunt has no valve. It lowers IOP by diverting aqueous humor from the anterior chamber into the subconjunctival space. One study found that the Ex-PRESS shunt lowered IOP by 40 percent in POAG patients who had the procedure. The shunt is reported to be easily inserted at the limbus (the very edge of the cornea, overlying the trabecular meshwork). Placement of the shunt is accomplished using a disposable inserter, after filling the anterior chamber with a viscoelastic material such as Viscoat or Healon.

Though the Ex-PRESS shunt is easily inserted, its insertion is a procedure that is most safely performed by an experienced glaucoma surgeon. Precise placement of the device is important in order to avoid touching the eye's lens and preventing the erosion of the implant through the conjunctiva overlying it. To reduce complications, glaucoma surgeons are studying the benefits of inserting this shunt under a scleral flap.

Because this device is so new, many glaucoma doctors are *very cautious* about its use and uncertain of its effectiveness, especially in the long term. The rates of complications are reportedly low in Europe, but have not yet been substantiated in the United States. Major concerns include hypotony (very low IOP), flat anterior chambers, bleeding, and erosion of the implant through the conjunctiva.

Much more study of this device is warranted to fully determine its safety and effectiveness.

# THE EYEPASS BIDIRECTIONAL GLAUCOMA IMPLANT

This glaucoma implant has been studied since 1999. It is a Y-shaped, tubular, silicone implant. It is constructed of two silicone tubes that are joined at one end. The device is inserted by dissecting through the sclera to Schlemm's canal. Once this canal is exposed, an opening is made. The tubular implant is inserted so that a portion of the device (equivalent of the upper portion of the Y) is inserted into the canal. The other part of the device is positioned so that its tip is inside the anterior chamber (the equivalent of the bottom part of the Y). Once the device is in place, aqueous first flows through the single tube that is within the anterior chamber. Aqueous continues along the device into one of the two tubes that are inside Schlemm's canal. IOP is lowered because aqueous outflow is increased. Essentially, aqueous is able to bypass the trabecular meshwork and flow directly out of the eye via Schlemm's canal. Studies of this device have follow-up of approximately two and a half years. These studies have found the IOP is reduced by 23 to 30 percent with 75 to 91 percent of patients reaching IOP levels of 21 mm Hg or lower.

The complication rate for this procedure is reportedly very low, with no hypotony or choroidal detachment. Further studies of this new glaucoma implant device are being performed.

# THE TRABECTOME

The trabectome is a new device that received FDA clearance in February 2004. It is a thin, probelike device that is inserted into the anterior chamber through a 1.5 mm corneal incision. The device has an insulated footplate that protects Schlemm's canal from damage while electrical energy is delivered to the trabecular meshwork. A system for irrigation is present on the device as well.

In this ten- to fifteen-minute procedure, the trabectome is passed into the anterior chamber through a small corneal incision. Once inside the anterior chamber, the device is viewed through a goniotomy lens and directed to the trabecular meshwork 180 degrees away from the entry site. The insulated footplate of the device is inserted into Schlemm's canal. Thermal energy is delivered by the trabectome to the trabecular meshwork in that area. A portion of the trabecular meshwork is ablated and stripped away while the footplate protects Schlemm's canal from being traumatized by the electrial energy being delivered by the device.

The trabectome, as currently being used, opens approximately thirty degrees of the trabecular meshwork. By applying thermal energy to the trabecular meshwork in this area, the resistance to outflow is reduced. Aqueous is more easily able to exit the eye via Schlemm's canal. As a result, IOP is lowered.

Although this device is new, initial results are promising. Complications include bleeding into the anterior chamber (hyphema) and corneal trauma. Further studies of this device are needed.

## ANTICIPATED IMPROVEMENTS IN SURGICAL TECHNIQUES

### Improved Cataract Removal

Surely the future will see improvements in the surgical techniques and instrumentation with which a cataract is removed. This new technology will have important implications for glaucoma patients who have cataract removal at the time of surgery to lower IOP (trabeculectomy).

## Specific Laser Phacoemulsification

One new surgical technique—called specific laser phaco-emulsification—is being developed and tested in clinical trials across the United States. Phacoemulsification, as we saw in chapter 9, is the procedure used in cataract removal surgery. The advantages of this new laser technique over the current standard, ultrasound, include a lack of heat generation and the requirement for only a very small incision (even smaller than with ultrasound phaco). In addition, new implants may be developed that can be injected through these very tiny incisions directly into the capsular bag. Specifically, this new technology will allow the length of the average clear corneal incision to be reduced from 2.75 to 1.8 millimeters. A smaller wound means more rapid healing and a lower complication rate.

As noted above, one advantage of laser phaco is its lack of heat generation while emulsifying the cataract lens. This lack of heat production may greatly reduce the occurrence of corneal burns. Researchers anticipate that phaco machines in the future will have both laser and ultrasound so that surgeons can use either or both techniques, depending on what the individual cataract surgery requires.

Laser phaco should also result in less inflammation and scarring. When cataract and glaucoma surgery are combined, it is important to have minimal inflammation. Laser phacoemulsification may help reduce the amount of inflammation during and after surgery.

Although the laser phaco looks promising and should improve the doctors' ability to perform cataract and glaucoma surgeries at the same time, it is generally believed that the standard for the *near future* will continue to be ultrasound phaco-emulsification.

## Aqualase

The new aqualase technology is a system in which heated saline solution is used to break up (soften and melt) the cataract. High-energy, high-velocity pulses of water break up the cataract material, which is then aspirated through a very small incision. Since neither laser nor ultrasound is used in this procedure, the risk of heat-related injury is even further reduced. Theoretically, aqualase will create less inflammation than ultrasound. Again, when used in combination with glaucoma surgery, reduced inflammation may improve success rates.

## Capsular Tension Rings

For patients with exfoliation syndrome, exfoliative glaucoma, and any other form of zonular weakness, the development of capsular tension rings is of great significance. Patients with these conditions often have weak zonules and unstable capsular bags. (You will recall that the capsular bag surrounds the eye's natural lens and that this bag is held in place by thousands of tiny fibers called zonules.) Zonular laxity and weakness predisposes the patient to a much greater complication rate during cataract removal surgery (phacoemulsification).

In patients with weakened zonules, the cataract may appear to have slight movements within the eye. This subtle movement indicates weak zonules and an unstable capsular bag. During cataract surgery, a capsular tension ring is inserted into the capsular bag to stabilize the bag and provide it with support. The device is available in multiple sizes. A larger ring is used when significant zonular or capsular bag weakness is detected.

Capsular tension rings were developed in the early 1990s but only recently became available in the United States. In the spring of 2004, the Food and Drug Administration approved a capsular tension ring called the Morcher capsular tension ring, a flexible, horseshoe-shaped filament with fixation eyelets at each end.

Patients who have weakened zonules and an unstable capsular bag should benefit in a significant way from the development of capsular tension rings—making cataract surgery in these patients much safer.

# Part IV

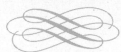

# AN "EYE" TOWARD THE FUTURE

# Chapter 15

# Genetics and Glaucoma

The importance of family history—and therefore, genetics—in glaucoma has been known for many years. Family history is one of the most significant risk factors for glaucoma. Whether you have any relatives with glaucoma is a question that every ophthalmologist will ask during a complete evaluation.

Too often, people are not even aware of their family medical histories of glaucoma. But such knowledge is vital because studies of families with glaucoma are among the key ingredients in the science of genetics. Researchers realize how important it is to study families with histories of glaucoma. They understand that this research will improve our understanding of the glaucomas, providing clues as to why and how the glaucomas occur.

The discovery of glaucoma-related genes has changed—and will continue to change—the way glaucoma is managed. Since the first glaucoma gene was discovered in 1997, researchers have found and confirmed at least eight glaucoma-related loci.

As more glaucoma genes are identified, the diagnosis, treatment, and prevention of glaucoma will be forever changed. Glaucoma will be diagnosed much more easily and earlier. Moreover, classification of the glaucomas will become more accurate. Specific underlying causes for each type of glaucoma will probably become known. Therapies will be tailored to an individual's specific type of glaucoma and its underlying genetic cause. Once doctors have identified the defective glaucoma gene for a specific type of glaucoma, gene therapy may be used. Gene therapy would replace the abnormal gene with a normal one before vision loss occurs.

The future will surely hold important breakthroughs based on information derived from today's research in the area of genetics. To achieve this, more research needs to be done. More families with glaucoma need to be studied.

One big problem that genetic scientists face in determining the genes that cause glaucoma is *genetic heterogeneity.* In addition to there being many different kinds of glaucoma, there are many different genes involved. Furthermore, different types of glaucoma may involve more than one gene. We have much to learn about the role each of them plays.

To identify each gene involved in every form of glaucoma, many families with glaucoma need to be studied. Clinicians need to ask these patients to take part in clinical studies, and patients need to agree to participate. Those who agree are usually referred to a genetics investigator. Small blood samples are drawn and sent to a genetics lab for analysis. Researchers then set out to link genetic mutations with certain markers, trying to estimate the location of the glaucoma gene(s).

## GENETIC LINKAGE

One key concept in understanding how genetics will help us is in the concept of *genetic linkage.* Genetic linkage looks for any links between the way a disease gene is inherited and the way a certain portion of DNA is inherited within a group of family members. When a link is found, this suggests that the gene being studied lies very close to the DNA segment that researchers already know.

After looking for linkage, researchers use genetic mapping to fine-tune the precise location of the gene. The gene is then cloned and sequenced. In this way, the function of a specific gene can be discovered.

## DISEASE-SPECIFIC GENETIC INFORMATION

### Juvenile Open-Angle Glaucoma (JOAG)

JOAG has been extensively studied in recent years. The condition has a dominant inheritance and an early age of onset. Researchers identified the first genetic location of a gene responsible for JOAG and called it GLC1A. (GLC1 is the label given for the open-angle disorders. The *A* is the label given for chromosome 1q25.) The discovery of GLC1A was accomplished by finding a large family with autosomal dominant JOAG and studying their genetics. (See the sidebar at the end of this chapter for definitions of some common genetics terms.) Researchers did numerous genetic tests on the family and found that their type of glaucoma was linked to a specific chromosome. This gene was called the myocilin or MYOC gene. The MYOC gene was localized to chromosome one. Myocilin could produce elevated intraocular pressure (IOP) by causing an obstruction of aqueous outflow through the trabecular meshwork. Recent studies show that the mutations in the myocilin gene are found in 10 percent of familial JOAG cases. Thus, scientists are concluding that more JOAG genes are yet to be discovered.

## Adult-Onset Primary Open-Angle Glaucoma (POAG)

Relative to JOAG, adult-onset OAG has a later age of onset and has less of a tendency to rapidly progress. Despite obvious differences between JOAG and adult-onset OAG, genetic studies show that these two types of glaucoma are sometimes not completely distinct. Some of their genetic makeup is the same. Genetic studies have also shown that there are myocilin (MYOC) gene mutations in almost 5 percent of patients with adult-onset OAG. In addition, researchers now know that other genes also contribute to adult-onset OAG, not just MYOC.

## Pigmentary Glaucoma and Pigmentary Dispersion Syndrome (PDS)

Genetic studies have shown that there is a dominant type of inheritance pattern in these disorders. Researchers have shown that *up to 50 percent of people with pigmentary dispersion syndrome go on to develop pigmentary glaucoma.* It is not known why certain individuals with PDS go on to develop pigmentary glaucoma and others don't, but genetic studies will help doctors learn why. The studies that have been done to date show that the myocilin gene (MYOC) is not involved in pigment dispersion syndrome. Clearly, further investigation (involving more and larger families) is required.

## Congenital Glaucoma

In congenital glaucoma, when a hereditary pattern is found, this pattern is usually autosomal recessive (requiring two copies of the gene mutation). In 1995, researchers studied seventeen families with autosomal recessive congenital glaucoma. These researchers were successful in identifying a genetic defect on chromosome GLC3A (2p21). (*GLC3* is the label for congenital forms of glaucoma.) A second genetic defect was discovered on chromosome GLC3B (1p36). It is believed that there is a third congenital glaucoma defect that has yet to be identified.

### Angle-Closure Glaucoma

In 1997, genetic researchers found that the gene 12q21 is associated with some forms of angle-closure glaucoma. In 1998, genetic researchers found a genetic linkage between angle-closure glaucoma and chromosome eleven. As with other forms of glaucoma, much work remains to be done.

### The OPAl Gene

One form of optic atrophy is inherited in a dominant fashion. This form of optic atrophy is called, therefore, autosomal dominant optic atrophy. Many genetic studies have been done on patients with this form of the disease. As a result, a gene on chromosome three was identified as being involved in the development of this disorder. This gene was named OPA1. Researchers hypothesize that the OPA1 gene may be involved with normal-tension glaucoma (NTG).

### Optineuron

At the time this book is being written, optineuron is the newest glaucoma gene to have been discovered. *Optineuron* stands for "optic neuropathy-inducing protein." This gene, though active throughout the entire body, is particularly involved with the workings of the trabecular meshwork, ciliary body, and the retina. Researchers discovered this gene when they were studying a large family with open-angle glaucoma.

When optineuron is abnormal, retinal ganglion cell death appears to occur more easily. When optineuron is not defective, it may provide neuroprotection to the optic nerve.

## FUTURE TARGETS FOR RESEARCH

Genetic research has made remarkable progress in the area of glaucoma. In the future, our understanding of the glaucomas will increase exponentially as more genetic studies are completed and more families with glaucoma are studied.

One recent breakthrough that will help genetic researchers is the completion of the Human Genome Project. In April 2003, the International Human Genome Sequencing Consortium completed its mapping of the entire human genetic code. With its completion, scientists are finding it easier to link diseases with their genetic defects. A more complete understanding of the glaucomas will follow.

In the future, gene therapy will play a very important role in glaucoma treatment. With gene therapy, doctors will be able to treat or target the trabecular meshwork itself and/or the parts of the eye that are involved with aqueous production. By treating or targeting these areas, IOP will be reduced or stabilized.

Gene therapy will do more than help lower or stabilize IOP. Though elevated IOP is the most commonly known and significant risk factor for glaucoma, there are other risk factors that are *not* related to elevated IOP. Examples of these include abnormally low blood pressure, migraines, Raynaud's syndrome, abnormal vascular autoregulation, sleep apnea, and autoimmune disease. These risk factors for the glaucomas may be treatable by gene therapy.

Some of the targets for gene therapy relate directly to apoptosis. As we know, the final common pathway for glaucoma is apoptosis—retinal ganglion cell death. Today's scientists are considering all the events that lead up to apoptosis to be targets for gene therapy. Optineuron, which may be a causative gene for normal-tension glaucoma, is another potential target for gene therapy.

## Delivery Systems

How would gene therapy be administered? Delivery systems will, by necessity, be tailored and very specific to glaucoma.

Targets for gene therapy in glaucoma patients would be any tissue or cell or structure that is involved with any part of the glaucomatous process. The most obvious examples include the trabecular meshwork, the ciliary body, and retinal ganglion cells, to name just a few.

The purpose of the delivery system is to effectively and safely deliver genes to the target. Often, viruses are used as such delivery vehicles. Examples of viral delivery systems include the adenoviruses and the herpes simplex viruses. An alternate delivery method is the injection of genetic material such as naked DNA into the eye. Researchers will surely consider the delivery of naked DNA to the anterior chamber in the treatment of glaucoma. This technique has already been used in the treatment of corneal disorders. Current research has shown that gene therapy can be delivered to the retinal ganglion cells through an injection into the vitreous. Future research will probably involve the delivery of gene therapy to the retina and ganglion cells by injecting the substance subretinally (below the retina). The beauty of this method is that the genes can be placed exactly where they are needed.

## Our Expectations for the Future

Researchers now believe that someday, gene therapy will allow doctors to control the production and outflow of aqueous, as well as prevent or slow the death of retinal ganglion cells.

Future research will concentrate heavily on trying to identify those genes that can lower IOP and protect retinal ganglion cells (neuroprotection). This type of gene therapy would prevent visual loss from glaucoma.

In the not-so-distant future, doctors will be able to order blood tests for genetic analysis that will yield tremendous information about an individual's specific type of glaucoma. Using that information, treatments will be meticulously tailored to that individual's genetic makeup. Furthermore, by knowing the details of a person's family history and that family's genetic makeup, the glaucoma risk for each member of the family will be more precisely determined and can be known before any glaucoma damage occurs.

Glaucoma doctors strongly believe that researchers *will* identify the causal genes for most specific types of glaucoma. Armed with that information, researchers will create new drugs that replace the defective proteins related to the glaucoma-inducing genes.

The National Institutes of Health have developed a database that is a catalog of human genes and genetic disorders. You can access the database at www.ncbi.nih.gov/omim/. For more information and referral to a genetics counselor see the resources section at the end of this book.

With the help of genetics and gene therapy, the goal of preventing glaucoma could become a reality in the near future.

## GENETIC TERMINOLOGY

There are some important genetic terms you need to understand as you learn more about genetics:

- **Autosomal dominant:** A trait that is expressed when only one copy of the gene is present.

- **Autosomal recessive:** A trait that is only expressed when two copies of the gene are present.

- **Chromosome:** A structure in the nucleus of a cell that contains a linear thread of DNA.

- **DNA (deoxyribonucleic acid):** A molecule that encodes genetic information in the nucleus of a cell.

- **Gene:** A biological unit of heredity; a segment of a DNA molecule that contains all the information required for the synthesis of a product.

- **Genetic mutation:** A gene in which the loss, gain, or exchange material has resulted in a permanent transmissible change in function.

- **Locus:** The site on a linkage map or chromosome where the gene for a particular trait is located.

- **Protein:** The principal constituent of the protoplasm of all cells, protein has a high molecular weight and consists essentially of combinations of amino acids in peptide linkages.

- **Sporadic:** Occurring occasionally, singly, or in scattered instances.

- **Trait:** A qualitative characteristic; a discrete attribute.

# Chapter 16

# New Directions: Protecting, Regenerating, and Replacing

Current therapy for glaucoma revolves around lowering intraocular pressure (IOP). But as I have discussed, IOP is just a risk factor for glaucoma—a *large* risk factor, but a risk factor nonetheless.

The future of glaucoma therapy includes medications and treatments that go beyond lowering IOP. Someday glaucoma patients will take eyedrops, pills, injections, or IV medications to help protect the optic nerve or allow it to regenerate. Patients with advanced vision loss may regain lost sight through retinal implants or replacement devices. Parts of the eye may be able to be regenerated through stem cell transplants.

These possibilities—and more—are some of the exciting new options being studied in glaucoma research centers across the country and around the globe.

# PROTECTING AND REGENERATING THE OPTIC NERVE

To find therapies to protect and regenerate the optic nerve, we must first understand how the cells become damaged and die as a result of glaucoma. A complete understanding of how retinal ganglion cells die is key. By understanding the details of retinal ganglion cell death (apoptosis), researchers will be able to determine ways in which this process can be modified or stopped.

## When Ganglion Cells Die

The steps involved with apoptosis are programmed into the cell when the cell is created. In other words, these complex steps are predetermined and genetically built-in. When a particular retinal ganglion cell receives the proper signal, a series of preprogrammed steps for cell death begin.

Research has already given us a number of theories of the steps that precede apoptosis. Some of these theories are:

- Blocked transport inside the axons.
- Loss of proper blood flow to the optic nerve head.
- Pressure on the retinal ganglion cells.
- And recently, the discovery that a neurotransmitter called glutamate is probably intimately involved in the steps that lead to apoptosis.

## Neuroregeneration

As you have learned in this book, the irreversible damage from glaucoma comes from the death of the retinal ganglion cell—the final common pathway in all glaucomas. In the near future, glaucoma therapy will include medications and treatments that protect these retinal ganglion cells. In the more distant future, it is hoped, glaucoma patients will be able to take medications that actually allow the optic nerve to *regenerate* and *reverse the damage.*

For most of us, the concept of neuroregeneration is the most exciting of all types of glaucoma research. The first step in learning how to regenerate retinal ganglion cell axons is to know how to keep the ganglion cell alive. In other words, researchers first need to find out how to save the retinal ganglion cells (that is, prevent them from undergoing apoptosis). Only a retinal ganglion cell that is *alive* can regenerate its axon!

In this regard, researchers are learning a lot from lower animals. Goldfish, for example, are able to regrow their axons and reconnect to the brain. Hopefully, the knowledge that researchers gain from studying the ways in which lower animals regenerate their own nerves will help researchers discover ways to help human retinal ganglion cells regenerate their axons.

In addition to studying goldfish and other lower animals, researchers are actively trying to understand the ways in which peripheral nerves regenerate. Peripheral nerves are those that do not connect directly to the brain—for instance, the nerves in your leg or hand. The optic nerve is a cranial nerve, which *does* connect directly to the brain. Researchers know that the regeneration of cranial nerves is a very different process from the regeneration of peripheral nerves. But researchers will be searching for any and all clues as to how the axons in cranial nerves can be encouraged to regenerate and reconnect. Also, glaucoma researchers will work closely with doctors studying spinal cord injuries and benefit from their efforts to understand and treat damaged nerve tissue.

Recently, researchers discovered that retinal ganglion cells are able to regenerate their axons to peripheral nerve grafts that are next to a cut optic nerve, but not into the optic nerve itself. Understanding this process is likely to provide scientists with a clearer understanding of neuroregeneration.

## Neuroprotection

Unfortunately, no proven neuroprotective drugs are currently available. But proven neuroprotective drugs *should* be a reality within the next several decades. Because researchers have a better understanding of how ganglion cells die in glaucoma (apoptosis), rapid progress in the development of neuroprotective drugs is expected.

Research today and in the future will involve a thorough examination and study of each of the steps involved in apoptosis. The scientists will be searching for ways to protect the optic nerve and the retinal ganglion cells. According to today's key glaucoma scientists, the three most likely strategies that researchers will be examining in the future include:

1. Preventing the initiation of apoptosis. (Don't let apoptosis start in the first place!)
2. Protecting retinal ganglion cells and their axons. (Could this protection come in the form of calcium channel blockers, antioxidants, immunization, or the blocking of glutamate receptors?)
3. "Rescuing" damaged axons and retinal ganglion cells. (Will this rescue be through antioxidants and/or nitric oxide synthase inhibitors?)

## The Role of Calcium

When retinal ganglion cells die, the amount of calcium inside the cell goes up significantly. These large increases in calcium (termed calcium influx) may contribute to retinal ganglion cell death. Brimonidine (Alphagan), an alpha-2 agonist, has been shown to have neuroprotective effects in studies of animals. Brimonidine has also been shown to block the influx of calcium. Betaxalol, a beta-blocker, has also been shown to have neuroprotective effects in recent animal studies, as well as to inhibit glutamate-receptor-stimulated increases in calcium within the retinal ganglion cells.

The role of calcium in neuroprotection is an area that will be studied closely in future research.

## The Role of Glutamate

Glutamate is an amino acid neurotransmitter. Humans and monkeys with glaucoma have higher than normal quantities of glutamate in their vitreous. Researchers will look at glutamate receptors and glutamate transporters to attempt to block the toxic effects of glutamate.

## Memantine: A Promising Drug

Memantine is the most exciting medication now being studied for neuroprotection. Currently used as a treatment for Parkinson's disease and Alzheimer's disease, Memantine is related to a Parkinson's medicine called amantadine.

Memantine is a glutamate receptor blocker. Glutamate receptors are intimately involved in stabilizing calcium inside a cell. Lack of oxygen in a cell, trauma to the optic nerve, and glaucoma all cause glutamate levels to rise significantly. High levels of glutamate are toxic to the nerve and are also associated with a very large increase of calcium within the neuronal cells. Calcium can trigger a series of events that ultimately leads to apoptosis. Researchers involved with memantine are trying to determine whether the drug can stop apoptosis by blocking these glutamate receptors. Allergan is conducting a multicenter, randomized clinical study examining the effects of memantine in patients with open-angle glaucoma. Researchers at Allergan are trying to determine whether the drug has a neuroprotective effect.

## The Role of Nitric Oxide (NO)

NO is a molecule involved in many functions in the body such as vasodilation, neuronal function, inflammation, and immune functions. NO is also involved in the regulation of apoptosis. It is generated by an enzyme called inducible nitric oxide synthase (iNOS). Researchers will be studying iNOS. If iNOS can be inhibited, then NO toxicity could be blocked.

## A Glaucoma Vaccine?

Dr. Michal Schwartz, a professor of neuroimmunology at the Weizmann Institute of Science in Rehovot, Israel, gained the world's attention with her dramatic new concept: a vaccine for glaucoma. This is among the most intriguing and exciting concepts on the horizon.

In 1996, Dr. Schwartz described glaucoma as a neurodegenerative disease. As such, glaucoma should be amenable to neuroprotective therapy. Dr. Schwartz made a number of crucial observations that have led to her theory about glaucoma and the concept of glaucoma vaccination:

- Elevated IOP is not the only cause of glaucoma damage. Many glaucoma patients develop further visual field loss despite a normal IOP.
- As glaucoma progresses, the disease itself contributes to the hostile conditions that cause it to worsen. For example, high levels of glutamate and nitric oxide have been found in patients with glaucoma.
- The cellular environments (substances inside and around

the cell) within the optic nerve influence their resistance to damage. For example, neurons that are capable of surviving might still die because of a slight increase in glutamate concentration.

- Today's knowledge of other degenerative diseases may be applicable to glaucoma.
- Finally, in 1999, Dr. Harry Quigley at Johns Hopkins established that the death of retinal ganglion cells in glaucoma (apoptosis) is a gradual process that involves changes within the cell that might be amenable to intervention.

Dr. Schwartz created a visionary concept of protective autoimmunity. Her concept envisions neuroprotection that is produced by enhancing part of the body's autoimmune response. By studying rats with chronic ocular hypertension (OHT), she found that vaccination can protect against the loss of retinal ganglion cells. Dr. Schwartz has described this type of therapy as one that boosts the body's own choice of therapy.

This groundbreaking research by Dr. Schwartz highlights an exciting function of the immune system—the ability to protect the body against its own self-destructive components.

## The Future of Neuroprotection

The discovery of neuroprotective medications is anxiously awaited by doctors and patients alike. It is an area of glaucoma research to which much energy and enthusiasm will be devoted in the near future. Still, difficulties and challenges in this research area lie ahead. Neuroprotection is difficult to measure and quantify. Moreover, studies of neuroprotection using animals may not apply to humans with glaucoma. The high doses of medicines and the ways of administering the study medications in animals may not be easily applied to humans. Furthermore, studies will require years to prove that a certain medication has neuroprotective effects. Despite these obstacles, however, it is clear that *the future of glaucoma therapy will combine treatments to lower IOP with medications or treatments to provide neuroprotection.* Someday, perhaps, neuroregeneration will also play a significant role in a glaucoma patient's care.

## RETINAL IMPLANTS

Currently, retinal implants are being developed to help patients blinded by retinitis pigmentosa and age-related macular degeneration (ARMD). *This technology may ultimately help patients who have lost sight related to glaucoma, but is of limited or no value in glaucoma patients whose optic nerve is severely damaged.*

The Doheny Retina Institute at the University of Southern California has developed the Model 1 epiretinal prosthesis. This device is reported to allow blind patients to see. The outer part of this device essentially consists of a camera, which is mounted on eyeglasses worn by the patient. The camera captures an image and digitizes it. This digital information is then transmitted wirelessly to a receiver inside the patient's eye. This receiver device is implanted on top of the retinal surface (epiretinal), not under the retina. When the digital, visual information is received by the device, the receiver delivers pulses of energy to the retinal neurons. These complex electrical charges are then transmitted through the optic nerve to the brain. The technology is similar to a cochlear implant for hearing.

The Model 1 epiretinal prosthesis allows patients to see movement and detect light and dark. The application of this or a related device to glaucoma is not known. It should also be noted that a device of this nature requires signals to be transmitted via the optic nerve to reach the brain. If the optic nerve is severely damaged by glaucoma, these signals may fail to be transmitted. The optic nerve may be unable to do the job.

## IMPLANTABLE MINIATURE TELESCOPE

VisionCare Ophthalmic Technologies in Saratoga, California, has developed a miniature telescope (approximately four millimeters long by three millimeters in diameter) that can actually be implanted in the eye of a person who has lost central vision due to age-related macular degeneration. The telescope is designed to replace the lens of the eye. It magnifies and projects objects over the portion of the retina that is undamaged. Though its application to glaucoma is questionable, this device may lead to a future device that will help glaucoma patients more effectively.

The advantage of this device over counterparts such as the retinal prosthesis is that it is placed entirely in the eye. As currently used, the eye surgeon implants the telescope in only one eye, which takes over central vision; the other eye takes over peripheral vision. The patient learns to adjust to the fact that each eye is seeing different views.

This very new technology is still in early clinical studies. However, early evidence indicates that it may prove useful in restoring sight to patients who had previously been functionally blind. Unfortunately, the benefits of this device in glaucoma may be severely limited or nonexistent. Once again, if the optic nerve has been too severely damaged by glaucoma, it will be unable to transmit the visual signals from this device to the brain.

## STEM CELL TRANSPLANTS

Another area of exciting research is stem cell transplantation. *Stem cells* are defined by the National Institutes of Health as cells that have the ability to divide for an indefinite period of time and give rise to specialized cells. Researchers believe that *stem cell therapy may offer the best hope for recovering vision that has already been lost to glaucoma.*

To date, this is just theory. Scientists do not yet hold all the keys to harvesting, differentiating, developing, and implanting stem cells. In terms of using stem cells to reverse glaucoma-induced damage to retinal ganglion cells, this technology may present extra problems. Not only do the cells need to survive and function, but they also need to form the proper connections with the brain for vision to be restored. Nevertheless, researchers believe that someday stem cells may become viable sources of replacement cells—even retinal ganglion cells!

Stem cell technology could be developed so the retinal ganglion cells that are destroyed in glaucoma could be replaced. This could reverse the blindness associated with the disease. Although such technology does not yet exist, stem cells could possibly grow new nerve tissue (including retinal ganglion cells) that could, in theory, be transplanted into the eyes of people who have lost vision. *Remarkably, with this technology, blindness from glaucoma could be reversed!*

# Part V

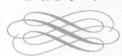

# WHAT YOU NEED
# TO KNOW NOW

# Chapter 17

# Protecting Yourself from the
# Sneak Thief of Sight

Glaucoma research holds great promise. New preventive measures, new treatments—even the reversal of blindness from glaucoma—all lie ahead. For now, however, early detection, meticulous monitoring, and diligent treatment remain the best ways to protect your sight.

Here's what you can do:

- If you have not been diagnosed with glaucoma, have yourself screened, or examined, regularly. How often you need to be checked depends on whether or not you fall into a high-risk category. If you are over age forty-five; of Asian, African, or Hispanic descent; have elevated intraocular pressure (IOP), diabetes, nearsightedness, or high (or low) blood pressure; have had a significant eye injury; have a history of long-term use of cortisone or steroids; or have a family history of glaucoma, *you should be examined by your eye doctor at least once per year* or according to your doctor's instructions.

- If you do not know (or are not sure) if you have a family history of glaucoma—*ask*! Don't forget to ask about glaucoma in aunts, uncles, and other more distant relatives. If you are diagnosed with glaucoma, make sure everyone in your family knows about it and understands that they may be at increased risk for developing the disease.

- If you are diagnosed with glaucoma, make sure you follow all your doctor's instructions. Talk with your doctor. Ask questions to better understand your glaucoma and its management. Take your medication exactly as prescribed; keep all your appointments for follow-up visits.

- Whether or not you are diagnosed with glaucoma, eat a diet rich in a variety of fruits and vegetables and keep your weight at a healthy level.

- Try to get at least thirty minutes of aerobic exercise four times per week.

- Stop smoking.

The future promises great advances in the diagnosis and treatment of glaucoma. Through research in genetics, doctors will be able to better predict who is most susceptible to developing glaucoma and develop new modes of treatment—and even prevention. Advanced diagnostic techniques will help doctors better detect and monitor glaucoma-related damage. New medications will provide enhanced benefits and fewer side effects. New surgical techniques will give us better ways to prevent and control glaucoma-related damage. Research in neuroprotection, regeneration, and transplantation will one day allow doctors to prevent or even reverse glaucoma-related damage to the optic nerve.

For now, however, the best defenses against "the sneak thief of sight" are regular examinations by your eye doctor, faithful compliance with your doctor's treatments, and the appropriate lifestyle changes. Eye examinations are especially important: The Glaucoma Foundation reminds us that 90 percent of all glaucoma-related blindness could have been prevented with proper treatment. But you can't get treated unless you know you have a problem.

The resources section of this book tells you where to go for additional information on glaucoma, other eye diseases, and low-vision assistance. You can also help others by supporting the research and patient education programs sponsored by charitable organizations such as The Glaucoma Foundation.

Sight is a precious gift that is worth protecting. See your eye doctor regularly. Learn more about glaucoma. Protect yourself and your loved ones from the sneak thief of sight.

## Appendix A

# Glaucoma and LASIK Surgery

Refractive surgery (such as LASIK) is the fastest-growing procedure in ophthalmology today. As LASIK grows in popularity, the issue of coexisting glaucoma becomes more important.

Since many of my glaucoma patients ask about LASIK, this book would not be complete without a short discussion of some of the most frequently asked questions and their answers.

### Is it safe to have LASIK if you have glaucoma?

To date, there has been no definitive study to determine the safety of LASIK in people with glaucoma. During the current LASIK procedure, a vacuum is placed on the eye in order to precisely cut a flap on the front surface of the cornea. While this vacuum is on, intraocular pressure (IOP) rises to 80 to 95 mm Hg. The typical amount of vacuum time is eleven seconds. With such a brief vacuum time, damage to the optic nerve or retinal nerve fiber layer (RNFL) is unlikely in a healthy patient. In the hands of an experienced LASIK surgeon, using minimal vacuum time, IOP-related damage is *not* probable. However, for a patient with glaucomatous cupping of the optic nerve head (disc) and visual field loss, LASIK should only be considered with great care and caution. For glaucoma patients, a lengthy discussion with your glaucoma doctor is a necessity before seriously considering a LASIK procedure.

## Is glaucoma more difficult to manage after LASIK?

Yes. During the LASIK procedure, the cornea is thinned. IOP measurement in an eye with a thinner cornea leads to an *underestimation* of the IOP. In a post-LASIK eye, an elevated IOP may be missed. It is important for all LASIK patients to inform their eye doctor that they had the LASIK procedure and remind the doctor that the IOP measurement may be an underestimation. Unfortunately, at present, there is no accepted conversion table to compute actual IOP for a cornea that is not of average thickness.

Second, patients who have undergone LASIK may require steroid eyedrops to control inflammation. These eyedrops, especially when required for lengthy periods of time, can raise IOP. This IOP elevation can be overlooked if IOP is underestimated and can be damaging to the optic nerve if it is significantly large.

## *Appendix B*

# Glaucoma and Pregnancy

Younger women with glaucoma are often worried about pregnancy and its effect on the management of their medical conditions and possible effects on their unborn child.

Women with glaucoma who are considering having children should discuss their situation with both their ophthalmologist and their obstetrician/gynecologist ... *before* they conceive. Since the greatest risk to the fetus occurs during the first trimester, it is best to plan ahead, before conception occurs. A woman may be pregnant for weeks before she even becomes aware of the pregnancy. She needs to discuss a plan to manage her glaucoma without medications with her doctors *at length* before proceeding with a pregnancy.

Some glaucoma medications are known to create adverse effects in animals. For obvious reasons, there have been no trials to determine potential adverse effects on the human fetus. None of the glaucoma medications has been tested on pregnant women. The potential risks of using glaucoma medications during the first trimester (and throughout the pregnancy) should be discussed with doctors, and a plan should be developed. A good possibility would be to minimize the exposure of the fetus to drugs during the first trimester. However, the risks associated with being off all glaucoma medications during the first trimester would need to be evaluated. This is *not* something a patient can or should decide on her own; decision making *with* the doctor is key.

Frequent monitoring of intraocular pressure (IOP) during this period is usually needed. If the patient's eye cannot tolerate an IOP elevation, surgery will probably be considered. Argon or selective laser trabeculoplasty (ALT or SLT) may allow the IOP to be adequately controlled without medications. Otherwise, glaucoma filtering surgery (trabeculectomy) would be considered.

If a pregnant woman must stay on glaucoma medications during her pregnancy, it is important that the nasolacrimal occlusion (NLO) technique be used to minimize the body's absorption of the medication. See the instructions for NLO in chapter 6.

Fortunately, there is no evidence that glaucoma has any impact on labor and delivery. In routine circumstances, IOP is not affected during labor and delivery. IOP *could* rise during periods of prolonged straining, but this would be temporary.

Nursing is another issue to discuss with the eye doctor, the obstetrician-gynecologist, and the pediatrician. Glaucoma medications do enter the circulation of the mother and could be secreted into her breast milk. In some instances, it may be advisable for a mother *not* to breast-feed her child while using glaucoma medications.

Overall, the management of glaucoma during pregnancy requires a team effort and open communication, with informed decision making that involves the patient and her doctors.

# *Appendix C*

## Glaucoma Medications

### Commonly Used Glaucoma Medications*

| Product/Brand Name | Generic Name | How Taken | How It Works | Major Side Effects |
|---|---|---|---|---|
| Alphagan (available only outside U.S.) | brimonidine 0.2% | 1 drop 2–3x/day | Reduces aqueous humor production, increases uveoscleral outflow | Allergic conjunctivitis, conjunctival redness, itchiness, stinging, dry mouth. |
| Alphagan P | brimonidine tartrate ophthalmic solution 0.15% | 1 drop 2–3x/day | Reduces aqueous humor production, increases uveoscleral outflow | Allergic conjunctivitis, conjunctival redness, itchiness, stinging, dry mouth. Purite as preservative has significantly reduced allergic symptoms relative to Alphagan. |
| Azopt | brinzolamide ophthalmic suspension 1% | 1 drop 2–3x/day | Reduces aqueous production | Blurred vision. Bitter, sour, or unusual taste. |
| Betagan | levobunolol hydrochloride ophthalmic solution, USP 0.5% | 1 drop 1x/day | Reduces aqueous production | Nonselective beta-blocker. See full list of associated side effects at end of chart.** Transient burning and stinging, blepharoconjunctivitis. |

| Product/Brand Name | Generic Name | How Taken | How It Works | Major Side Effects |
|---|---|---|---|---|
| Betoptic S | betaxolol HCL 0.25% | 1 drop 2x/day | Reduces aqueous production | Selective beta-blocker. Selective beta-blockers have fewer pulmonary side effects than nonselective beta blockers. See full list of associated side effects at end of chart.** Transient ocular discomfort. |
| Cosopt | dorzolamide hydrochloride-timolol maleate ophthalmic solution | 1 drop 2x/day | Reduces aqueous production | All side effects of Trusopt or timolol are possible. See full list of side effects associated with nonselective beta-blockers at end of chart.** Taste perversion, ocular burning and/or stinging, conjunctival redness, blurred vision, or eye itching. |
| Daranide | dichlorphenamide 50 mg tablets | Priming dose of 2 to 4 tablets, followed by 2 tablets every 12 hours until desired response is attained; recommended maintenance dose is ½ to 1 tablet 1–3x/day | Reduces aqueous production | Headache, malaise, fatigue, lethargy, nausea, vomiting, diarrhea, poor appetite, taste alteration, metabolic acidosis, electrolyte imbalance, reduced potassium, tingling of fingers and toes, kidney stones, frequent urination. |

| Product/Brand Name | Generic Name | How Taken | How It Works | Major Side Effects |
|---|---|---|---|---|
| Diamox and Diamox Sequels sustained-release capsules | acetazolamide 500 mg (Sequels) or 125 or 250 mg (tablets) | Up to 1000 mg per day in divided doses | Reduces aqueous production | Headache, malaise, fatigue, lethargy, nausea, vomiting, diarrhea, poor appetite, taste alteration, metabolic acidosis, electrolyte imbalance, reduced potassium, tingling of fingers and toes, kidney stones, frequent urination. |
| Epifrin | epinephrine, USP 0.5%, 1.0%, and 2.0% | 1 drop 1–2x/day | Reduces aqueous inflow and increases aqueous outflow | Eye pain or ache, brow ache, headache, hypertension, blurred vision, macular edema, conjunctival redness, and allergic lid reaction. |
| Iopidine | apraclonidine 0.5% and 1.5% | 1 drop 2x/day (often used before lasers to blunt IOP spikes) | Reduces aqueous humor production, increases uveoscleral outflow | Redness, allergy, pupillary dilation, dry mouth, dry eye, hypotension, lethargy. Avoid if using MAO inhibitors. |
| IsoptoCarbachol | carbachol 0.75%, 1.5%, and 3.0% | 1 drop 3x/day | Increases aqueous outflow | Blurred/dim vision, cataract, increased redness, retinal detachment, brow ache, accommodative spasm. |
| Lumigan | bimatoprost ophthalmic solution 0.03% | 1 drop 1x/day (usually bedtime) | Increases outflow of aqueous through trabecular meshwork and uveoscleral routes | Redness, eyelash growth, iris pigmentation changes, darkening of eyelids, burning, stinging, irritation. Associated with more redness than other hypotensive lipids. |

| Product/Brand Name | Generic Name | How Taken | How It Works | Major Side Effects |
| --- | --- | --- | --- | --- |
| Neptazane | methazolamide 25 and 50 mg tablets | Maximum dose: 50 mg 3x/day | Decreases production of aqueous | Headache, malaise, fatigue, lethargy, nausea, vomiting, diarrhea, poor appetite, taste alteration, metabolic acidosis, electrolyte imbalance, reduced potassium, tingling of fingers and toes, kidney stones, frequent urination. |
| Ocupress | carteolol hydrochloride ophthalmic solution USP, 1% | 1 drop 2x/day | Reduces aqueous production | Nonselective beta-blocker. See full list of associated side effects at end of chart.** Transient eye irritation, burning, tearing, conjunctival redness and puffiness. Less bradycardia than other beta-blockers. |
| OptiPranolol | metipranolol ophthalmic solution 0.3% | 1 drop 2x/day | Decreases aqueous production | Nonselective beta-blocker. See full list of associated side effects at end of chart.** Transient local discomfort. |
| Phospholine Iodide | echothiophate iodide 0.03% 0.06%, 0.125%, and 0.25% | 1 drop 2x/day | Increases aqueous outflow | Stinging, burning, lacrimation, lid muscle twitching, conjunctival and ciliary redness, brow ache, induced myopia, visual blurring. |
| Pilocar | pilocarpine 1–8% | 1 drop 4x/daily | Increases aqueous outflow | Blurred/dim vision, cataract, increased redness, retinal detachment, brow ache. |
| Pilopine HS gel | pilocarpine 4% | Into eye at bedtime | Increases aqueous outflow | Blurred/dim vision, cataract, increased redness, retinal detachment, brow ache. |

| Product/Brand Name | Generic Name | How Taken | How It Works | Major Side Effects |
|---|---|---|---|---|
| Propine | dipivefrin hydrochloride 0.1% | 1 drop 2x/day | A pro-drug of epinephrine; decreases aqueous production and enhances outflow facility | Same as epinephrine, but less systemic side effects since it is a pro-drug. Redness, burning, stinging, allergic symptoms, blurred vision. Increased heart rate, palpitations. |
| Rescula | unoprostone isopropyl ophthalmic solution 0.15% | 1 drop 2x/day | Increases uveoscleral outflow | Redness, eyelash growth, iris pigmentation changes, darkening of eyelids, burning, stinging, irritation. |
| Timoptic (also available in Ocudose dispenser); also available as Betimol | timolol maleate ophthalmic solution 0.25% and 0.5% | 1 drop 2x/day | Decreases production of aqueous | Nonselective beta-blocker. See full list of associated side effects at end of chart.** Burning and stinging upon instillation. |
| Timoptic-XE sterile Ophthalmic gel-forming solution and timolol GFS | timolol maleate ophthalmic gel-forming solution 0.25% and 0.5% | 1 drop 1x/day (usually A.M.) | Decreases production of aqueous | Nonselective beta-blocker. See full list of associated side effects at end of chart.** Because this drug is dosed only once a day, the body is exposed to less medication and there are fewer bodily side effects than with twice-a-day timolol. Transient blurred vision, pain, redness, discharge, foreign-body sensation, itching, and tearing. |

| Product/Brand Name | Generic Name | How Taken | How It Works | Major Side Effects |
|---|---|---|---|---|
| Travatan | travoprost ophthalmic solution 0.004% | 1 drop 1x/day (usually bedtime) | Increases uveoscleral outflow | Redness, eyelash growth, iris pigmentation changes, darkening of eyelids, burning, stinging, irritation. |
| Trusopt | dorzolamide hydrochloride ophthalmic solution 2% | 1 drop 2–3x/day | Decreases aqueous production | Burning, stinging, or discomfort immediately following administration; bitter taste following administration. |
| Xalatan | latanoprost ophthalmic solution 0.005% | 1 drop 1x/day (usually bedtime) | Increases uveoscleral outflow | Redness, eyelash growth, iris pigmentation changes, darkening of eyelids, burning, stinging, irritation. Macular edema, including cystoid macular edema. |
| Xalcom (available only outside U.S.) or Xalacom | latanoprost ophthalmic solution 0.005% and timolol 0.5% | 1 drop 1x/day | Increases uveoscleral outflow and decreases aqueous production | All side effects seen in Xalatan plus those of timolol. |

*Please note that generic versions of some of these products exist, but are too numerous to list.

**Common systemic side effects associated with beta-blockers include low blood pressure, low heart rate, difficulty breathing, fatigue, weakness, decrease in exercise tolerance, insomnia. Uncommon side effects include decreased libido, depression, weakness, impotence, hair loss.

# Glaucoma Medications Administered by Physicians in Emergency Situations

(For Patients with Extremely Elevated IOP)

| Product/Brand Name | Generic Name | How Taken | How It Works | Major Side Effects |
|---|---|---|---|---|
| Glycerol, Glyrol, Osmoglyn | Glycerine (oral) 50% solution | 1.0–1.5 g/kg of body weight (orally) | Osmotic agent that decreases vitreous volume; carbohydrate (lasts up to 5 hours) | Serious metabolic abnormalities, especially in diabetics. |
| Ismotic | Isosorbide (oral) 50% solution | 1.0–1.5 g/kg of body weight (orally) | Osmotic agent that decreases vitreous volume; excreted in urine unmetabolized (effects last 3–5 hours) | Fewer metabolic disturbances. Safer than Glycerol for diabetics. |
| Mannitol, Osmitrol | 20% IV solution | Given intravenously (1–2 gm/kg of body weight) over 30 minutes | Osmotic agent; decreases vitreous volume (effects last up to 6 hours) | Renal failure, congestive heart failure, headache, angina-like pain, pulmonary edema. |

# Glossary

**Alpha-2 agonists:** A class of glaucoma medications that increase the drainage of aqueous from the eye *and* decrease the rate at which aqueous is produced within the eye, thereby lowering IOP. Examples: Alphagan P, brimonidine.

**Amblyopia:** "Lazy eye."

**Angle:** The structures within the area where the iris meets the cornea. Also refers to the specific way in which the iris meets the cornea.

**Anterior chamber:** The space in the eye that is behind the cornea and in front of the iris and pupil.

**Antimetabolite:** An antiscarring agent used in conjunction with glaucoma filtration surgery.

**Apoptosis:** Programmed cell death.

**Aqualase:** A new technology being developed for cataract removal.

**Aqueous humor:** The watery substance produced by the ciliary body that provides the cornea and lens with nutrients and oxygen and helps maintain the necessary pressure for the eye to retain its shape. Also simply called aqueous.

**Aqueous shunt:** An implantable device in which a small tube extends into the anterior chamber. The tube is connected to one or more plates that are sutured to the surface of the eye. Aqueous drains through this shunt and lowers IOP.

**Argon laser iridoplasty (ALI):** A laser procedure performed to contract the tissue at the extreme periphery of the iris, closest to the drain, enhancing drainage of aqueous by further opening the angle.

**Argon laser trabeculoplasty (ALT):** A procedure in which an argon laser light is applied to trabecular meshwork to improve the flow of aqueous through the drain.

**Autoimmune diseases:** Diseases in which the body's immune system attacks itself or specific organs or tissues of the body.

**Autosomal dominant:** A trait that is expressed when only one copy of the gene is present.

**Autosomal recessive:** A trait that is only expressed when two copies of the gene are present.

**Axon:** A neuron's appendage that transmits signals away from the cell body.

**Beta-blockers:** For glaucoma, a class of medications that decrease the rate at which aqueous is produced by the eye, thereby lowering IOP.

**BID:** Twice a day.

**Bilateral:** Relating to both eyes.

**Bleb:** A small, cystlike elevation created on the surface of the eye during trabeculectomy. The reservoir into which aqueous drains before being reabsorbed by the body's venous system.

**Carbonic anhydrase inhibitors:** A class of glaucoma medications that decrease the rate at which aqueous is produced within the eye.

**Central retinal vein occlusion (CRVO):** Blockage in the central retinal vein.

**Central vision:** "Straight-ahead" vision.

**Cholinergic agents:** A class of glaucoma agents that increase the drainage of aqueous from the eye. Example: pilocarpine.

**Choroid:** The vascular middle coat of the eye, positioned between the sclera and retina.

**Choroidal effusion:** Buildup of fluid in the choroidal system.

**Chromosome:** A structure in the nucleus of a cell that contains a linear thread of DNA.

**Ciliary body:** The structure that produces the aqueous humor.

**Confocal scanning laser ophthalmoscopy (CSLO):** The technology used in Heidelberg Retinal Tomographs (HRT) to quantitatively analyze the optic nerve head and related structures.

**Conjunctiva:** A semitransparent tissue that contains many blood vessels and covers the surface of the eyeball.

**Conjunctivitis:** "Pinkeye." An inflammation of the conjunctiva, often viral or bacterial or allergic in origin.

**Cornea:** The clear, outer portion of the eye, through which light enters.

**Corneal edema:** When the cornea becomes swollen with fluid.

**Correctopia:** When the pupil becomes decentered.

**Cryotherapy:** Treatment with extreme cold, freezing tissues. It is used commonly to treat an ischemic retina, and also to damage the ciliary body, thereby reducing aqueous production and lowering IOP.

**Cup:** The pale, central zone of the optic nerve head.

**Cup-to-disc ratio:** The size of the cup relative to the disc.

**Cupping:** When the cup-to-disc ratio is greater than normal.

**Cyclodestructive procedures:** Procedures that reduce IOP by damaging the ciliary body, causing a reduction in the amount of aqueous produced.

**Dilate:** The use of eyedrops to enlarge the pupil, allowing a better view of the structures in the back of the eye, such as the retina and optic nerve head.

**Disc:** A reddish "saucer" around the cup on the optic nerve head.

**Diurnal curve:** A record of IOP levels over time—usually hourly over an entire day.

**DNA (deoxyribonucleic acid):** A molecule that encodes genetic information in the nucleus of a cell.

**Drift:** The phenomenon by which glaucoma medications gradually lose their effectiveness over time.

**Endophthalmitis:** A type of very serious eye infection involving the inside of the eye.

**Episcleral venous pressure (EVP):** Pressure in the veins (located in the connective tissue between the sclera and the conjunctiva) that drain aqueous after it passes through the trabecular meshwork.

**Epithelial downgrowth:** A condition in which epithelial cells (which normally lie on the outside of the eye) grow inward onto structures inside the eye, often blocking the trabecular meshwork.

**ERG:** An objective test of retinal function.

**5-Fluorouracil (5-FU):** An antimetabolite that is injected beneath the conjunctiva after glaucoma filtration surgery to prevent or slow scar tissue formation.

**Frequency doubling technology (FDT):** A form of visual field testing that is often used in glaucoma screening.

**Gene:** A biologic unit of heredity; the segment of a DNA molecule that contains all the information required for synthesis of a product.

**Genetic mutation:** A gene in which the loss, gain, or exchange of material has resulted in a permanent transmissible change in function.

**Glaucomatous optic neuropathy:** A specific type of damage to the optic nerve.

**Ghost cells:** Cells formed when red blood cells from a hemorrhage inside the eye break down.

**Goldmann tonometry:** A test in which the physician measures the patient's IOP by touching a small instrument (attached to the slit lamp) to the corneal surface of the eyeball.

**Gonioplasty:** A procedure in which laser energy is applied to the iris closest to the trabecular meshwork (drain). The laser spots cause the iris tissue to contract and pull away from the drain. As the iris pulls away, the drain is reopened and aqueous is able to enter.

**Goniopuncture (laser):** A procedure in which the YAG laser is used to make an opening in the membrane that separates the filter from the anterior chamber following nonpenetrating glaucoma filtering surgery (if IOP is insufficiently lowered by the surgery).

**Gonioscope:** A mirrored lens that enables doctors to view the angle of the eye.

**Gonioscopy:** The examination of the anterior chamber of the eye (including the trabecular meshwork) using a gonioscope.

**Heidelberg Retinal Tomograph (HRT):** A device that provides three-dimensional quantitative analysis of the optic nerve head topography.

**Heterochromia irides:** Different-colored irides between two eyes of the same person.

**Humphrey perimetry:** A visual field test using a Humphrey perimeter (usually white-on-white stimuli).

**Hyperemia:** Redness of the eye.

**Hyphema:** Blood in the anterior chamber of the eye.

**Hypotensive lipids:** Glaucoma medications that increase the drainage of aqueous from the eye. There are two types of hypotensive lipids: prostaglandin analogs and prostamide compounds.

**Hypotony:** Abnormally low IOP.

**IOP:** Intraocular pressure—pressure within the eyeball.

**IOL:** Intraocular lens—an artificial lens implanted during cataract surgery.

**Iridodenesis:** A condition in which the iris moves, shakes, and quivers easily.

**Iris:** The pigmented portion of the eye that is visible through the clear cornea (plural: *irides*).

**Iris bombé:** "Bowing" forward of the iris.

**Iritis:** Inflammation of the iris and anterior chamber.

**Ischemia:** A condition in which inflow of blood is obstructed, causing a lack of oxygen to the tissue.

**Krukenberg Spindle (K Spindle):** A narrow, vertical, spindle-shaped deposit of pigment on the innermost surface of the cornea, seen in pigmentary glaucoma.

**Laser:** A highly concentrated and powerful beam of light used in eye (as well as other) surgeries. The term is an acronym for "light amplification by stimulated emission of radiation."

**Laser peripheral iridectomy:** A term sometimes used to describe laser peripheral iridotomy. Although both terms are technically correct, this book uses *laser peripheral iridotomy* to describe the procedure.

**Laser peripheral iridotomy (LPI):** A procedure in which laser energy is used to make an opening through the iris, allowing aqueous to move easily from the posterior chamber into the anterior chamber. It is used in narrow- or closed-angle conditions.

**Laser suture lysis:** A procedure to cut a suture that has been placed onto the eye during trabeculectomy, thereby increasing aqueous outflow and reducing IOP.

**Laser trabecular ablation:** A nonpenetrating glaucoma filtration procedure.

**Laser trabeculoplasty:** A laser procedure in which laser energy is applied to the trabecular meshwork to improve aqueous outflow and lower IOP.

**LASIK:** A type of refractive surgery using an excimer laser.

**Lens:** The eye's crystalline structure that lies immediately behind the iris. The lens variably focuses for the eye.

**Locus:** The site on a linkage map or chromosome where the gene for a particular trait is located.

**Macrophages:** "Scavenger" cells that remove debris.

**Macula:** The area in the center of the retina that provides the clearest sight.

**Macular edema:** Swelling in the central area of the retina.

**Metabolite:** The active form of a pro-drug.

**Miotic drops:** Eyedrops that constrict the pupil and are used to lower IOP. Example: pilocarpine.

**Monotherapy:** Treatment with only one medication.

**Myocilin (MYOC):** The gene for juvenile open-angle glaucoma. The first glaucoma gene discovered, located on chromosome one. It has many mutations.

**Myopia:** Nearsightedness.

**Nasolacrimal occlusion (NLO):** A technique involving the application of gentle pressure on the inner corner of the eye by the tear duct after the instillation of an eye drop in order to maximize the medicine's absorption by the eye and minimize the absorption by the body.

**Needling of the bleb:** A surgical procedure in which the doctor attempts to revive a failing (or poorly functional) filtration bleb. This is done by using instruments to break the superficial scar tissue within the filtration site that is blocking outflow of aqueous.

**Neuroprotective effect:** The ability of a medication or therapy to protect the optic nerve from damage, independent of its IOP-lowering effect on the eye.

**Nodules:** Tiny, pigmented bumps or elevations.

**Nonpenetrating glaucoma surgery:** Surgery that creates a glaucoma filter without entering the eye.

**Ocular hypertension (OHT):** Elevated IOP without damage to the optic nerve or visual field (without signs of glaucoma).

**Ophthalmoscope exam:** An exam in which the doctor looks inside the eye and visualizes the optic nerve.

**Optic disc hemorrhages:** Small hemorrhages on the surface or edge of the optic nerve head.

**Optic nerve:** The cranial nerve (analogous to a massive cable) that transmits the signals and impulses received by the retina to the brain.

**Optic nerve head:** The very top of the optic nerve that can be visualized by the eye doctor when looking into the eye.

**Optical coherence tomography (OCT):** A technology that produces cross-sectional images of the retina.

**Optineuron:** Optic neuropathy-inducing protein.

**Pallor:** Pale coloration.

**Paracentesis:** A tiny opening into the anterior chamber through the cornea used to reinflate the front chamber of the eye during trabeculectomy or release aqueous from the anterior chamber to reduce IOP temporarily.

**Patent:** Open.

**Penetrating keratoplasty (PK):** Corneal transplant.

**Peripapillary:** Next to the disc.

**Peripheral anterior synechiae (PAS):** Scar tissue that seals the iris onto and often over the trabecular meshwork, blocking the flow of aqueous out of the eye.

**Peripheral iris:** Tissue at the extreme periphery of the iris, closest to the drain.

**Peripheral vision:** To-the-side vision.

**Phaco:** Abbreviation for *phacoemulsification*.

**Phacodenesis:** A condition in which the lens moves, shakes, and quivers easily.

**Phacoemulsification (phaco):** A surgical procedure for cataract removal (most commonly using ultrasound).

**Phaco-trab:** Combined cataract–glaucoma (trabeculectomy) surgery.

**Phagocytes:** Cells that eat and remove debris and pigment.

**Plateau iris configuration:** The peripheral iris appears to be bent sharply forward so the iris lies extremely close to the trabecular meshwork, while the central iris plane is flat.

**Pneumotonometer (pneumatic tonometer):** A pencil-shaped instrument that measures IOP by using air or gas to determine the force required to flatten the cornea.

**Posterior chamber:** The portion of the eye that lies between the iris and the lens.

**Posterior sclerostomy:** A surgical procedure in which a small opening is made in the back part of the sclera to allow fluid—which would normally be trapped in the choroid—to escape the eye.

**Posterior subcapsular cataract (PSC):** A type of cataract in which the back layers of the lens are most affected and are most cloudy. This type of cataract is often seen in eyes exposed to steroids and/or inflammation. Symptoms are blurred vision, glare, and poor reading vision.

**Presbyopia:** The reduced ability to focus near objects, generally occurring as people reach ages forty to forty-five.

**Pro-drug:** A drug that is inactive while in the bottle but converted to an active form as it enters the eye.

**Prostaglandin analog:** A type of hypotensive lipid. Examples: Xalatan, Travatan.

**Prostamide compound:** A type of hypotensive lipid. Example: Lumigan.

**Protein:** The principal constituents of the protoplasm of all cells.

**Pupil:** The central aperture of the iris through which light enters the eye.

**QD:** Once a day.

**Retina:** An inner layer of the eye; it contains the nerve cells that capture and transmit images to the optic nerve.

**Retinal ganglion cells:** Nerve cells within the retina that are destroyed in glaucoma.

**Retinal thickness analyzer (RTA):** An instrument that can image the optic disc and measure retinal thickness in the macula and peripapillary regions.

**Retrobulbar tumors:** Tumors behind the eye.

**RNFL:** Retinal nerve fiber layer.

**Sampolesi's Line:** The "line" of pigment deposited on the surface of the angle, common in patients with exfoliation syndrome.

**Scanning laser polarimetry (SLP):** A technology that allows doctors to image the optic nerve head and quantitatively evaluate the retinal nerve fiber layer that lies adjacent to it.

**Schlemm's canal:** A channel contiguous with the trabecular meshwork. The traditional route of outflow for the aqueous humor.

**Sclera:** Thick, outer shell of the eye.

**Selective laser trabeculoplasty (SLT):** A procedure in which YAG laser light (instead of argon laser) is applied to the trabecular meshwork to improve the flow of aqueous through the drain.

**Short wavelength automated perimetry (SWAP):** A highly sensitive visual field test that uses blue dots of light on a yellow background instead of the standard white on white.

**Slit lamp:** An instrument (a microscope with a high-intensity light source) used to examine the various structures of the eye.

**Sporadic:** Occurring occasionally, singly, or in scattered instances. Occurring randomly.

**Swedish interactive thresholding algorithm (SITA):** A visual field test algorithm (program) that provides reliable and accurate information in a relatively brief period of time and customizes the visual field for each individual patient.

**Sympathomimetics:** A class of glaucoma medications that increase the drainage of aqueous from the eye. Example: Propine.

**Tonometer (Goldmann):** An instrument (attached to the slit lamp) that measures IOP.

**Tonometer (noncontact):** A device that uses a puff of air to measure IOP.

**Tonometer (Proview):** A device for at-home, self-monitoring of IOP.

**Tonometer (Schiotz):** A portable tonometer that requires the patient to be lying down, faceup.

**Tono-Pen:** A small, portable, pencil-shaped device that measures IOP by indenting the cornea and calculating the electrical signal generated.

**Trabecular meshwork:** The part of the eye that functions as a drain.

**Trabeculectomy:** Filtering surgery that increases the outflow of aqueous, lowering IOP.

**Trabeculitis:** Inflammation of the trabecular meshwork.

**Trait:** A qualitative characteristic; a discrete attribute.

**Unilateral:** Relating to one eye only.

**Uvea:** A highly vascular area consisting of the choroid, ciliary body, and iris.

**Uveitis:** Inflammation of the uvea.

**Viscocanalostomy:** A form of nonpenetrating surgery.

**Visual field:** The area of vision, including central vision and peripheral vision. By monitoring a patient's visual field, the doctor can determine whether vision is being lost.

**Visual evoked response (VER):** The electrical response generated in response to a specific stimulation of the retina. Also called visual evoked potential (VEP).

**Visual field test:** A test in which the patient is asked to detect flashes of light to determine whether any vision has been lost, especially peripheral (side) vision.

**Vitrectomy:** Surgery in which the vitreous (or part thereof) is removed.

**Vitreous humor:** The gel-like substance that fills the area behind the lens. Also referred to as simply the vitreous.

**Zonules:** Thousands of tiny fibers that hold the crystalline lens in place behind the iris.

# Resources

Please consult my Web site for the most up-to-date patient and clinical information on glaucoma: www.GregoryHarmonMD.com.

The following organizations and their Web sites can provide you with additional information about glaucoma.

**The Glaucoma Foundation**
80 Maiden Lane
Suite 1206
New York, NY 10038
212-285-0080
info@glaucomafoundation.org
www.glaucomafoundation.org

The Glaucoma Foundation runs several online support communities that patients and families find especially helpful: Young and Under Pressure (YUP, for teens and young adults under thirty); YUP Parents; and Adult Patients Under Pressure.

**American Glaucoma Society**
P.O. Box 193940
San Francisco, CA 94119

415-561-8587
ags@aao.org
www.glaucomaweb.org

## American Academy of Ophthalmology
P.O. Box 7424
San Francisco, CA 94120-7424
415-561-8555
eyemd@aao.org
www.aao.org

## The Glaucoma Research Foundation
490 Post Street
San Francisco, CA 94102
800-826-6693
415-986-3162
info@glaucoma.org
www.glaucoma.org

## Prevent Blindness America
500 East Remington Road
Schaumburg, IL 60173
888-331-2020
info@preventblindness.org
www.preventblindness.org

## National Association for Visually Handicapped
22 West 21st Street
New York, NY 10011
212-889-3141
staff@navh.org
www.navh.org

## Lighthouse International
111 East 59th Street
New York, NY 10022-1202
212-821-9200

info@lighthouse.org
www.lighthouse.org

**National Eye Institute**
31 Center Drive, MSC 2510
Bethesda, MD 20892-2510
301-496-5248
www.nei.nih.gov

**The American Board of Medical Specialties**
866-ASK-ABMS (275-2267)
Call this number to confirm that your eye doctor is board certified.

# GENETICS RESOURCES

## LABORATORIES OFFERING
## RESEARCH TESTING FOR GLAUCOMA

**Duke University Medical Center**
**Center for Human Genetics**
  Durham, NC
  John Gilbert, PhD; Margaret Pericak-Vance, PhD; Marcy
  C. Speer, PhD; Jeffrey M. Vance, MD, PhD; Michelle
  Winn, MD
  Director: Margaret Pericak-Vance, PhD
  Primary contact: Bob Broomer, CCRP
  800-422-1575
  919-681-6585
  broom002@mc.duke.edu
  Primary contact: Jennifer Caldwell
  800-422-1575
  919-681-2746
  caldw018@mc.duke.edu

Laboratory accepts contact from patients/families.

**University of Michigan Kellogg Eye Center**
**Glaucoma Genetics Laboratory**
  Ann Arbor, MI
  Julia E. Richards, PhD
  Director: Julia E. Richards, PhD
  Genetic counselor: Catherine A. Downs, MS, CGC
  734-936-7384
  downs@umich.edu
Laboratory accepts contact from health care providers only.

## FOR REFERRAL TO A GENETIC COUNSELOR

**National Society of Genetic Counselors Executive Office**
233 Canterbury Drive
Wallingford, PA 19086-6617
610-872-7608
www.nsgc.org/resourcelink.asp

**Online Mendelian Inheritance in Man (OMIM)**
www.ncbi.nlm.nih.gov/entrez/query.fcgi?db-OMIM/
Online catalog of human genes and genetic disorders.
Authored and edited by Dr. Victor A. McKusick and
colleagues. Developed for the Internet by the National
Center for Biotechnology Information, National Institutes
of Health.

# How You Can Help

Do you want to help advance glaucoma research and enhance public outreach and patient education for glaucoma? Consider a contribution to one of the following organizations. No amount is too small to make a difference.

**The Glaucoma Foundation**
80 Maiden Lane
Suite 1206
New York, NY 10038
212-285-0080

**The Cornell Glaucoma Fund**
c/o June Maldonado-Resto
Weill-Cornell Medical College
520 East 70th Street
Starr Pavilion 823
New York, NY 10021
212-746-2475

# References

## JOURNALS AND PERIODICALS

Age-Related Eye Disease Study Research Group. A Randomized, placebo-controlled, clinical trial of high-dose supplementation with vitamins C and E, beta-carotene, and zinc for age-related macular degeneration and vision loss. AREDS report no. 8. *Arch Ophthalmol.* 2001; 119(10):1417–1436.

Age-Related Eye Disease Study Research Group. A randomized, placebo-controlled clinical trial of high dose supplementation with vitamins C and E, beta-carotene for age-related cataract and vision loss: AREDS report no. 9. *Arch Ophthalmol.* 2001; 119(10)1439–52.

AGIS Investigators. The advanced glaucoma intervention study (AGIS): 4. Comparison of treatment outcomes within race. Seven-year results. *Ophthalmology.* 1998; 105(7)1146–64.

AGIS Investigators. The advanced glaucoma intervention study: 9. Comparison of glaucoma outcomes in black and white patients within treatment groups. *Am J Ophthalmol.* 2001;132(3):311–20.

Avunduk AM, Yilmaz B, Sahin N, et al. The comparison of intraocular pressure reductions after isometric and isokinetic exercises in normal individuals. *Ophthalmologica.* 1999;213(5):290–4.

Aydin P, Oram O, Akman A, Dursan D. Effect of wind instrument playing on intraocular pressure. *J Glaucoma.* 2000;9(4):322–4.

Bain WES, Maurice DM. Physiological variations in the intraocular pressure. *Trans Ophthalmol Soc UK.* 1959;79:249–60.

Barràs T, Brandt CR, Nickells R, Ritch, R. Gene therapy for glaucoma: Treating a multifaceted, chronic disease. *Invest Ophthalmol Vis Sci.* 2002:43(8):2513–18.

Beatty S, Koh H.-H, Phil M, et al. The role of oxidative stress in the pathogenesis of age-related macular degeneration. *Surv Ophthalmol.* 2000;45:115–134.

Bengtsson B, Heijl A. Comparing significance and magnitude of glaucomatous visual field defects using the SITA and Full Threshold strategies. *Acta Ophthalmol.* 1999;77:143–146.

Bengtsson B, Heijl A. Evaluation of a new perimetric threshold strategy, SITA, in patients with manifest and suspect glaucoma. *Acta Ophthalmol.* 1998;76:268–72.

Bengtsson B, Heijl. Inter-subject variability and normal limits of the SITA Standard, SITA Fast, and the Humphrey Full Threshold computerized perimetry strategies, SITA STATPAC. *Acta Ophthalmol Scand.* 1999;77:125–129.

Bengtsson B, Olsson J, Heijl A, et al. A new generation of algorithms for computerized threshold perimetry, SITA. *Acta Ophthalmol.* 1997;75:368–375.

Bigger JF. Glaucoma with elevated episcleral venous pressure. *South Med J.* 1975;68:1444–8.

Bonomi L, Marchini G, Marraffa M, Bernardi P, Morbio R, Varotto A. Vascular risk factors for primary open angle glaucoma: the Egna-Neumarkt Study. *Ophthalmology.* 2000;107:1287–1293.

Booth FW, Gordon SE, Carlson CI, et al. Waging the war on modern chronic diseases: primary prevention through exercise biology. *J Appl. Phys.* 2000;88:774–87.

Bovell, A, Damji, MD. Understanding glaucoma from the inside out. *Geriatric Ophthalmology.* December 2002, 10–12.

Buono LM, Foroozan R, Sergott RC, et al. Is normal tension glaucoma actually an unrecognized hereditary optic neuropathy? New evidence from genetic analysis. *Current Opinion in Ophthalmol.* 2002;13(6):362–70.

Brandt JD. The influence of corneal thickness on the diagnosis and management of glaucoma. *J Glaucoma.* 2001;10:S65–67.

Brandt JD, Beiser JA, Kass MA, Gordon MO. Central corneal thickness in the Ocular Hypertension Treatment Study (OHTS). *Ophthalmology.* 2001;108(10):1779–1788.

Britt MT, LaBree LD, Lloyed MA. Randomized clinical trial of 350 mm2 versus the 500 mm2 baerveldt implant: longer terms results: Is bigger better? *Ophthalmology.* 1999;106(2):2312–18.

Brown, Linda J. Alternative therapies for glaucoma. *Eye World.* 2003;8(4):97.

Brubaker RF et al. Guide to glaucoma management: A continuing medical education program. *Rev Ophthalmology.* September 2001.

Bruttini M, Longo I, Frezzotti P, et al. Mutations in the myocilin gene in families with primary open angle glaucoma and juvenile open angle glaucoma. *Arch Ophthalmol.* 2003;121(7):1034–38.

Chandler P. Long-term results of glaucoma therapy. *Am J Ophthalmol.* 1960;49:221–246.

Cho E, Hankinson SE, Willett WC, et al. Prospective study of alcohol consumption and the risk of age-related macular degeneration. *Arch Ophthalmol.* 2000;118(5):681–8.

Cho E, Hung S, Willett WC, et al. Prospective study of dietary fat and the risk of age-related macular degeneration. *Am J Clin Nutr.* 2001;73(2):209–18.

Cho E, Stampfer MJ, Seddon JM, et al. Prospective study of zinc intake and the risk of age-related macular degeneration. *Ann Epidemiol.* 2001;11(5):328–36.

Chung HS, Harris A, Kristinsson JK, et al. Ginkgo biloba extract increases ocular blood flow velocity. *J Ocul Pharmacol Ther.* 1999;15(3):233–40.

Cimberle, Michela. Research on retinal implants progresses. *Ocular Surgery.* January 15, 2003. p 74.

Coleman AL. Glaucoma. *Lancet.* 1999;354(9192):1803–10.

Coleman AL, Mondino BJ, Wilson MR, Casey R. Clinical Experience with the Ahmed Glaucoma Valve Implant in eye with prior or concurrent penetrating keratoplasties. *Am J Ophthalmol.* 1997; 123:54–61.

Collaborative Normal-Tension Glaucoma Study Group. Comparison of glaucomatous progression between untreated patients with normal-tension glaucoma and patients with therapeutically reduced intraocular pressures. *Am J Ophthalmol.* 1998:126:487–505.

Collaborative Normal-Tesion Glaucoma Study Group. The effectiveness of intraocular pressure reduction in the treatment of normal-tension glaucoma. *Am J Ophthalmol.* 1998;126(4):498–505.

Damji, KF, Allingham, RR. Molecular Genetics is revolutionizing our understanding of ophthalmic disease. *Am J Ophthalmol* 1997;124:530–543.

Damji KF, Muni FH, Munger FM. Influence of corneal variables on accuracy of intraocular pressure measurement. *J Glaucoma.* 2003; 12(1):69–80.

Doughty MJ. Human corneal thickness and its impact on intraocular pressure measures: a review. *Surv Ophthalmol.* 1994; 29:73–6.

Drance S, Anderson DR, Schulzer M. Collaborative Normal-Tension Glaucoma Study Group. Risk factors for progression of visual field abnormalities in normal-tension glaucoma. *Am J Ophthalmol.* 2001;131:699–708.

DuBiner H, Cooke D, Dirks M, et al. Efficacy and safety of bimatoprost in patients with elevated intraocular pressure: A 30-day comparison with latanoprost. *Surv Ophthalmol.* 2002;45(suppl 4):S353–S360.

Ehlers N, Bramson T, Sperling S. Applanation tonometry and central corneal thickness. *Acta Ophthalmol.* 1975;53:34–43.

Ehlers N, Jhortdal J. Corneal thickness; measurement and implications. *Exp Eye Res.* 2004 Mar, 78(3):543–8. Review.

Evans JR. Antioxidant vitamin and mineral supplements for age-related macular degeneration. *Cochrane Database Syst Rev.* 2002;2:CD000254.

Feuer WJ, Parrish RK, Schiffman JC, et al. The ocular hypertension treatment study: Reproducibility of cup/disk ratio measurements over time at an optic disc reading center. *Am J Ophthalmol.* 2002;133:19–28.

Fingeret M, Flanagan JG. Repeatability of the Proview Eye Pressure Monitor. Presented at Association for Research in Vision and Ophthalmology (ARVO), Fort Lauderdale, FL. May 2003. Presentation 2178.

Gandolfi SA, Cimino L. Effect of bimatoprost on patients with primary open-angle glaucoma or ocular hypertension who are non-responders to latanoprost. *Ophthalmology.* 2003;110(3)609–614.

Gandolfi S, Simmons ST, Sturm R, et al. The Bimatoprost study Group 3. Three-month comparison of bimatoprost and latanoprost in patients with glaucoma and ocular hypertension. *Adv Ther.* 2001;18:110–121.

Garcia-Feijoo J, Duran-Poveda S, Cuina-Sardina R, et al. Ultrasound biomicroscopy of an implantable miniaturized telescope. *Arch Ophthalmol.* 2001;119(10):1544–6.

Ghandi P, Gurses-Ozden R, Liebmann J, et al. Attempted eyelid closure affects intraocular pressure measurement. *Am J Ophthalmol.* 2001;131:417–420.

Goldberg J, Flowerdew G, Smith E, et al. Factors associated with age-related macular degeneration. An analysis of data from the first National Health and Nutrition Examination Survey. *Am J Epidemiol.* 1988;128(4):700–10.

Goldberg L, Elliot DL, Van Buskirk, EM. Exercise training reduces intraocular pressure among subjects suspected of having glaucoma. *Arch Ophthalmol.* 1991;109:1096–1098.

Gordon MO, Beiser JA, Brandt JD, et al. The Ocular Hypertension Treatment Study: baseline factors that predict the onset of primary open-angle glaucoma. *Arch Ophthalmol.* 2002.120:714–720.

Haynes WL, Johnson AT, Alward WL. Effects of jogging exercise on patients with the pigmentary dispersion syndrome and pigmentary glaucoma. *Ophthalmology.* 1992;99(7):1096–103.

Hayreh SS, Podhajsky P, Zimmerman MB. Role of nocturnal hypertension in optic nerve head ischemic disorders. *Ophthalmologica.* 1999:213:76–96.

Head, KA. Natural therapies for ocular disorders, part two: cataracts and glaucoma. *Altern Med Rev.* 2001;6(2):141–66.

Heijl A, Leske MC, Bengtsson B, et al. Reduction of intraocular pressure and glaucoma progression: results from the Early Manifest Glaucoma Trial. *Arch Ophthalmol.* 2002;120:1268–79.

Heijl A, Bengtsson B, Patella VM. Glaucoma follow-up when converting from long to short perimetric threshold tests. *Arch Ophthalmol.* 2000;118:489–493.

Herndon LW, Weizer JS, Stinett SS. Central corneal thickness as a risk factor for advanced glaucoma damage. *Arch Ophthalmol.* 2004;122(1):17–21.

Herndon L, et al. Central corneal thickness in normal, glaucomatous, and ocular hypertensive eyes. *Arch Ophthalmol.* 1997;115: 1137–1141.

Herndon LW, Weizer JS, Stinnett SS. Central corneal thickness as a risk factor for advanced glaucoma damage. *Arch Ophthalmol.* 2004;122:17–21.

Heuer DK, Lloyed Ma, Abrams DA, et al. Which is better? One or two? A randomized clinical trial of single-plate versus double-plate Molteno implantation for glaucomas in aphakia and pseudophakia. *Ophthalmology.* 1992;99:1512–19.

Higginbotham EJ, Schuman JS, Goldberg I, et al. One-year, randomized study comparing bimatoprost and timolol in glaucoma and ocular hypertension. *Arch Ophthalmol.* 2002;120(10):1286–93.

Hitchings R. Intraocular pressure and circulation at the disc in glaucoma. *Acta Ophthalmologica Scandinavia.* 1997;15–22.

Hodkin MJ, Goldblatt WS, Burgoyne CF, Ball SF. Early clinical experience with the Baerveldt Implant in complicated glaucomas. *Am J Ophthalmol.* 1995;120:32–40.

Huang MC, Netland PA, Coleman AL, et al. Intermediate-term clinical experience with the Ahmed Glaucoma Valve implant. *Am J Ophthalmol.* 1999;127(1):27–33.

Hughes E, Spry P, Diamond J. 24-Hour monitoring of intraocular pressure in glaucoma management: A retrospective review. *J Glaucoma.* 2003;12(3):232–6.

Ishida K, Yamamoto T, Suglyama K, Kitazawa Y. Disk hemorrhage is a significantly negative prognostic factor in normal-tension glaucoma. *Am J Ophthalmol.* 2000;129:707–714.

Jamal KN, Gurses-Ozden R, Liebmann JM, et al. Attempted eyelid closure affects intraocular pressure measurement in open-angle glaucoma patients. *Am J Ophthalmol.* 2002;134:186–9.

Jay JL, Allan D. The benefit of early trabeculectomy versus conventional management in primary open angle glaucoma relative to severity of disease. *Eye.* 1989;8:528–535.

Johnson EJ. The role of lutein in disease prevention. *Nutrition in Clinical Care.* 2000;3:289–296.

Kalant H. Medicinal use of cannabis: history and current status. *Pain Res Manag.* 2001 Summer;6(2)80–91.

Kaluza G, Strempel I, Maurer H. Stress reactivity of intraocular pressure after relaxation training in open-angle glaucoma patients. *J Behav Med.* 1996;19(6):587–98.

Kano K, Kuwayama Y, Mizoue S. Clinical results of selective laser trabeculoplasty. *Acta Societatis Ophthalmol Japan.* 1999;103(8):612–6.

Karger RA, Jeng SM, Johnson DH. Estimated incidence of pseudoexfoliation syndrom and pseudoexfoliation glaucoma in Olmsted County, Minnesota. *J Glaucoma.* 2003;12(3):193–7.

Karmel, Miriam. New perimetry devices promise earlier detection. *Eyenet.* October 2002. 19–20.

Kass MA, Heuer DK, Higginbotham EJ, et al. The Ocular Hypertension Treatment Study Group. The Ocular Hypertension Treatment Study: a randomized trial determines that topical ocular hypotensive medication delays or prevents the onset of primary open-angle glaucoma. *Arch Ophthalmol.* 2002;120:701–713.

Kelker AE. Visual prognosis in advanced glaucoma: a comparison of medical and surgical therapy for retension of vision in 101 eyes with advanced glaucoma. *Trans Am Ophthalmol Soc.* 1977;75:539:555.

Kennan AM, Mansergh FC, Fingert JH, et al. A novel Asp 380 Ala mutation in the GLC1A/myocilin gene in a family with juvenile onset primary open-angle glaucoma. *J Med Genetics.* 1998;35(11):957–60.

Kinkead, Gwen. Stem cell transplants offer hope in some cases of blindness. *The New York Times.* April 15, 2003. F7.

Klein BE, Klein R, Jensen SC. Open-angle glaucoma and older-onset diabetes. The Beaver Dam Eye Study. *Ophthalmology.* 1994;101:1173–1177.

Klein BE, Klein R, Meuer SM, Goetz LA. Migraine headache and its association with open-angle glaucoma: the Beaver Dam Eye Study. *Invest Ophthalmol Vis Sci.* 1993;34:3024–3027.

Klein BE, Klein R, Sponsel WE, et al. Prevalence of glaucoma. The Beaver Dam Eye Study. *Ophthalmology.* 1992;99(10):1499–504.

Kobayashi H, Kobayashi K, Okinami S. A comparison of intraocular pressure-lowering effect of prostaglandin F2-[alpha] analogues, latanoprost, and unoprostone isopropyl. *J Glaucoma.* 2001;10(6):487–92.

Kosoko O, Quigley, HA, Vitale S, et al. Risk factors for noncompliance with glaucoma follow-up visits in a residents' eye clinic. *Ophthalmology.* 1998;105:2105–2111.

Kountouras J, Myolpoulos N, Chatzopoulos C, et al. Eradication of Helicobacter pylori may be beneficial in the management of chronic open-angle glaucoma. *Arch Intern Med.* 2002;162(11):1237–44.

Lafuente MP, Villegas-Perez MP, Sobrado-Calvo P, et al. Neuroprotective effects of alpha(2)-selective adrenergic agonists against ischemia-induced retinal ganglion cell death. *Invest Ophthalmol Vis Sci.* 2001;42(9):2-74-84.

Lakhanpal RR, Yanai D, Weiland JD, et al. Advances in the development of visual prostheses. *Current Opinion in Ophthalmol.* 2003;14(3):122–7.

Latina MA, Sibayan SA, Shin DH, et al. Q-switched 532-nm Nd:YAG laser trabeculoplasty (selective laser trabeculoplasty): a multicenter, pilot, clinical study. *Ophthalmology.* 1998;105(11)2082–8.

Lebowitz HM, Krueger DE, Maunder LR, et al. The Framingham Eye Study monograph: An ophthalmological and epidemiological study of cataract, glaucoma, diabetic retinopathy, macular degeneration, and visual acuity in a general population of 2631 adults, 1973–1975. *Surv Ophthalmol.* 1980;24(Suppl):335–610.

Lee AJ, Rochtchina E, Wang JJ, et al. Does smoking affect intraocular pressure: Findings from the Blue Mountains Eye Study. *J Glaucoma.* 2003;12:209–212.

Leske MC, Connell AM, Wu SY, Hyman LG, Schachat AP. Risk factors for open-angle glaucoma. The Barbados Eye Study. *Arch Ophthalmol.* 1995;113:918–924.

Leske MC, Heijl A, Hussein M, et al. Factors for glaucoma progression and effect of treatment. The Early Manifest Glaucoma Trial. *Arch Ophthalmol.* 2003; 121:48–54.

Leske MC, Heijl A, Hyman L, et al. Early manifest glaucoma trial: design and baseline data. *Ophthalmology.* 1999; 106:2144-53.

Lichter PR, Musch DC, Gillespie BW, et al. Interim clinical outcomes in the Collaborative Initial Glaucoma Treatment Study comparing initial treatment randomized to medications or surgery. *Ophthalmology.* 2001;108(11)1943–1953.

LiJ, Herndon LW, Stinnett S, Asrani SG, Allingham RR. Clinical comparison of the Proview Eye Pressure Monitor with Goldmann Applanation Tonometer and Tono-Pen. Presented at Association for Research in Vision and Ophthalmology, May 2003. Presentation 79.

Lin, S. Endoscopic cyclophotocoagulation. *Br J Ophthalmol.* 2002;86:1434–8.

Linden C, Alm A. Acetylsaliclic acid does not reduce the intraocular pressure variation in ocular hypertension or glaucoma. *Exp Eye Res.* 2000;70(3):281–3.

Lloyd MA, Baerveldt G, Fellenbaum PS, et al. Intermediate term results of a randomized clinical trial of the 350 versus the 500 mm Baerveldt Implant. *Ophthalmology.* 1994;101:1256–64.

Manzi F, Flood V, Webb K, Mitchell P. The intake of carotenoids in an older Australian population: The Blue Mountains Eye Study. *Public Health Nutrition.* 2002;5:347–352.

Mao LK, Steward WC, Shields MB. Correlation between intraocular pressure control and progressive glaucomatous damage in primary open-angle glaucoma. *Am J Ophthalmol.* 1991;111(1):51–5.

Mark HH. Corneal curvature in applanation tonometry. *Am J Ophthalmol.* 1973;76:223–4.

McDonnell PJ, Robin JB, Schanzlin DJ, et al. Molteno Implant for control of glaucoma in eyes after penetrating keratoplasty. *Ophthalmology.* 1988;95:364–9.

Melmed S, Cahane M, Gutman I. Blumenthal M. Postoperative complications after Molteno Implant surgery. *Am J Ophthalmol.* 1991;1:319–22.

Mermoud A, Salmon JF, Straker C, Murray AND. Use of the single plate molteno implant in refractory glaucoma. *Ophthalmologica.* 1992;205:113–120.

Mojon DS, Hess CW, Goldblum D, et al. High prevalence of glaucoma in patients with sleep apnea syndrome. *Ophthalmology.* 1999;106:1009–1012.

National Eye Institute of the National Institutes of Health, Statement on Glaucoma and Marijuana Use, February 18, 1997.

National Eye Institute of the National Institutes of Health, Statement on Age-Related Macular Degeneration and Wine Consumption, May 1998.

National Eye Institute of the National Institutes of Health, Statement on Lutein and its Role in Eye Disease Prevention, July 2002.

Netland PA, Landry T, Sullivan K, et al. Travaprost compared with latanoprost and timolol in patients with open-angle glaucoma or ocular hypertension. *Am J Ophthalmol.* 2001;132(4):472–84.

Netland PA, Robertson SM, Sullivan EK, et al. Response to travoprost in black and nonblack patients with open-angle glaucoma or ocular hypertension. *Advances in Therapy.* 2003;20(3):149–63.

Neufeld A, et al. Inhibition of nitric-oxide synthase 2 by aminoguanidine provides neuroprotection of retinal ganglion cells in a rat model of chronic glaucoma. *Proc Natl Acad Sci.* 1999;17;96:9944–8.

Noecker RS, Dirks MS, Choplin NT et al. A six-month randomized clinical trial comparing the IOP-lowering efficacy of bimatoprost and latanoprost in patients with oocular hypertension or glaucoma. *Am J Ophthalmol.* 2003;135:55–63.

Nyska A, Glovinsky Y, Belkin M, Epstein Y. Biocompatibility of the Ex-PRESS miniature glaucoma drainage implant. *J Glaucoma.* 2003;12:275–280.

Obisesan TO, Hirsch R, Kosoko O, et al. Moderate wine consumption is associated with decreased odds of developing age-related macular degeneration in NHANES-1. *J Am Geriatr Soc.* 1998; 46(1):114.

Parrish R, Palmberg P. Sheu W. A comparison of latanoprost, bimatoprost and travoprost in patients with elevated intraocular pressure: A 12-week, randomized, masked-evaluator multicenter study. *Am J Ophthalmol.* 2003;135:688–703.

Partamian LG, Lee DA, Ryan T, et al. Miniature continuous intraocular pressure sensor. Paper presented at: Annual meeting of the Association for Research in Vision and Ophthalmology; May 6, 2003; Fort Lauderdale, Florida.

Passo MS, Goldberg L, Elliot DL, Van Buskirk EM. Exercise training reduces intraocular pressure among subjects suspected of having glaucoma. *Arch Ophthalmol.* 1991;109(8):1096–8.

Piechocki, Michael. Rate of retinal complications following refractive surgery depends on procedure. *Ocular Surgery.* January 15,2003. 77–8.

Piltz J, Gross R, Shin DH, et al. Contralateral effect of topical beta-adrenergic antagonists in initial one-eyed trials in the Ocular Hypertension Treatment Study. *Am J Ophthalmol.* 2000;130(4):441–453.

Plasilova M, Stoilov I, Sarfarazi M, et al. Identification of a single ancestral CYP1B1 mutation in Slovak gypsies (Roms) affected with primary congenital glaucoma. *J Med Genetics.* 1999;36(4):290–4.

Pradalier A, Hamard P, Sellem E, Bringer L. Migraine and glaucoma: an epidemiologic survey of French ophthalmologists. *Cephalalgia.* 1998;18:74–76.

Preferred Practice Pattern: Primary Open-Angle Galucoma. American Academy of Ophthalmology 2000.

Purcell JJ, Tillery W. Hair glaucoma (corresp). *Arch Ophthalmol.* 1973;89:530.

Quigley HA. The search for glaucoma genes—implications for pathogenesis and disease detection. *New England J Med.* 1998;338(15)1063–4.

Racette L, Wilson MR, Zangwill LM, et al. Primary open-angle glaucoma in blacks: a review. *Surv Ophthalmol.* 2003;48(3):295–313.

Rafuse PE, Mills DW, Hooper PL, et al. Effects of Valsalva's manoeuver on intraocular pressure. *Can J Ophthalmol.* 1994;29:73–6.

Rai S, Moster MR, Kesen M, et al. Preview of Proview—Evaluation of the home tonometer. Presented at Association for Research in Vision and Ophthalmology (ARVO), Ft. Lauderdale Florida, May 2003. Presentation 4346.

Rezaie T, Child A, Hitchings R, et al. Adult onset primary open angle glaucoma caused by mutations in Optineuron. *Science.* 2002;295:1077–1079.

Rhee DJ, Katz LJ, Spaeth GL, Myers JS. Complementary and alternative medicine for glaucoma. *Surv Ophthalmol.* 2001 Jul–Aug; 46(1):43–55.

Rhee DJ, Spaeth GL, Myers, JS, et al. Prevalence of the use of complementary and alternative medicine in glaucoma. *Ophthalmology.* 2002;109(3):438–43.

Ritch R. Potential role for Ginkgo biloba extract in the treatment of glaucoma. *Med Hypotheses.* 2000;54(2):221–35.

Ritch R, Reyes A. Moustache glaucoma (corresp). *Arch Ophthalmol.* 1988;106:1505.

Scerra, Chet. Genetic research provides greater understanding of OAG. *Ophthalmology Times.* April 1, 2003. 29–31.

Schneemann A, Leusink-Muis A, van den Berg T, et al. Elevation of nitric oxide production in human trabecular meshwork by increased pressure. *Graefe's Arch Clin Exp Ophthalmol.* 2003;241:321–326.

Schuman JS, Massicotte EC, Connolly S, et al. Increased intraocular pressure and visual field defects in high resistance wind instrument players. *Ophthalmology.* 2000 Jan;107(1)127–33.

Schwartz M. Harnessing the immune system for neuroprotection: therapeutic vaccines for acute and chronic neurodegenerative disorders. *Cell Mol Neurobiol.* 2001;21(6):617–27.

Sekhar GC, Naduvilath TJ, Lakkai M, et al. Sensitivity of Swedish Interactive Threshold Algorithm Compared with Standard Full Threshold Algorithm in Humphrey Visual Field Testing. *Ophthalmology.* 2000;9:20–27.

Sharma AK, Goldberg I, Graham SL, et al. comparison of the Humphrey Swedish Interactive Thresholding Algorithm (SITA) and Full Threshold strategies. *J Glaucoma.* 2000;0:20–27.

Sherwood M, Brandt J. Bimatoprost Study Groups 1 and 2. Six month comparison of bimatoprost once-daily and twice-daily with timolol twice-daily in patients with elevated intraocular pressure. *Surv Ophthalmol.* 2001:45(suppl4):S361–8.

Shily BG. Psychophysiological stress, elevated intraocular pressure, and acute closed-angle glaucoma. *Am J Optom Physiol Opt.* 1987;64(11):866–70.

Shingleton BJ, Richter CU, Dharma SK, et al. Long-term efficacy of argon laser trabeculoplasty. A 10-year follow-up study. *Ophthalmology.* 1993;100(9):1324–9.

Shirato S, et al. A new family of perimetric testing strategies. *Graefe's Arch Clin Exp Ophthalmol.* 1999;237:29–34.

Singh K, Spaeth G, Zimmerman T, Minckler D. Target pressure—glaucomatologists' holy grail. *Ophthalmology.* 2000;107(4):629–630.

Stephenson, Michelle. Aqualase comes of age and supporters welcome its rise. *Eyeworld.* December 2002. 18.

Stone EM, Fingert JH, Alward WL, et al. Identification of a gene that causes primary open angle glaucoma. *Science.* 1997;275 (5300):668–70.

Teng C, Gurses-Ozden R, Liebmann JM, Tello C, Ritch R. Effect of a tight necktie on intraocular pressure. *Br J Ophthalmol.* 2003;87: 946–948.

Tielsch JM, Sommer A, Katz J, et al. Racial variations in the prevalence of primary open-angle glaucoma. The Baltimore Eye Survey. *JAMA.* 1991;266(3):369–74.

Tsai, JC, Johnson, CC, Dietrich, MS. The Ahmed shunt versus the Baerveldt shunt for refractory glaucoma. *Ophthalmology.* 2003;110(9):1814–21.

The AGIS Investigators. The Advanced Glaucoma Intervention Study (AGIS):7. The relationship between control of intraocular pressure and visual field deterioration. *Am J Ophthalmol.* 2000;130(4):429–440.

The AGIS Investigators. The Advanced Glaucoma Intervention Study (AGIS): 11. Risk factors for failure of trabeculectomy and argon laser trabeculoplasty. *Am J Ophthalmol.* 2002;134(4):481–498.

The Fluorouracil Filtering Surgery Study Group. Fluorouracil Filtering Surgery Study three-year follow-up. *Am J Ophthalmol.* 1993;115:82–92.

The Glaucoma Laser Trial Research Group: The Glaucoma Laser Trial 1. Acute effects of argon laser trabeculoplasty on intraocular pressure. *Arch Ophthalmol.* 1989;107:1135–42.

The Glaucoma Laser Trial Research Group: The Glaucoma Laser Trial 2. Results of argon laser trabeculoplasty versus topical medicines. *Ophthalmology.* 1990;97:1403–13.

The Ocular Hypertension Study. *Arch Ophthalmol.* 2002;120: 701–713.

Wang JJ, Mitchell P. Smith W. Is there an association between migraine headache and open-angle glaucoma? Findings from the Blue Mountains Eye Study. *Ophthalmology.* 1997;104:1714–1719.

*Weizmann Institute of Science Annual Report.* Battling glaucoma. 2002. 10–11.

Whitacre MM, Stein R. Sources of error with use of Goldmann-type tonometers. *Surv Ophthalmol.* 1993;38:1–30.

Wild JM, et al. The SITA perimetric threshold algorithms in glaucoma. *Invest Ophthalmol Vis Sci.* 1999;1998–2009.

WoldeMussie E, Yoles E, Schwartz M, et al. Neuroprotective effect of memantine in different retinal injury models in rats. *J Glaucoma.* 2002;11(6):474–80.

Wong TY, Klein BE, Klein R, Knudtson M, Lee KE. Refractive errors, intraocular pressure, and glaucoma in a white population. *Ophthalmology.* 2000;110(1):211–7.

Wunder, H. A new number in the glaucoma equation. *Rev Ophthalmol.* June, 2003:41–43.

Yoles E, Schwartz M. Elevations of intraocular glutamate levels in rats with partial lesion of the optic nerve. *Arch Ophthalmol.* 1998;116(7):906–10.

Yu D-Y, Morgan WH, Su E-N, et al. Robotic biological microfistula implantation for glaucoma drainage surgery (a preliminary report). Paper presented at: Annual meeting of the Association for Research in Vision and Ophthalmology; May 6, 2003; Fort Lauderdale, Florida.

Zeyen T. Target pressures in glaucoma. *Bull Sec Belge Ophthalmol.* 1999;274:61–65.

## CONFERENCE CATALOGS AND
## UNPUBLISHED MATERIALS

*GLAUCOMA TRIALS AND TRIBULATIONS*
American Academy of Ophthalmology
Subspecialty Day (in conjunction with the
American Glaucoma Society) November 15, 2003

Allingham, RR. Genetic testing for glaucoma: Are we there yet? *Glaucoma Trials and Tribulations.* American Academy of Ophthalmology. 2003:73–76.

Brandt, JD. Does every patient in a glaucoma practice require measurement of corneal thickness? Yes. *Glaucoma Trials and Tribulations.* American Academy of Ophthalmology. 2003:39–42.

Burgoyne, CF. Retinal nerve fiber layer assessment: Past, present, and future. *Glaucoma Trials and Tribulations.* American Academy of Ophthalmology. 2003:45–49.

Chauhan, BC. Is there a role for Frequency Doubling Technology? *Glaucoma Trials and Tribulations.* American Academy of Ophthalmology. 2003:7–8.

Cioffi, GA. Does every patient in a glaucoma practice require measurement of corneal thickness? No. *Glaucoma Trials and Tribulations.* American Academy of Ophthalmology. 2003:43.

Crandall, AS. The two-site cataract-trabeculectomy combined procedure. *Glaucoma Trials and Tribulations.* American Academy of Ophthalmology. 2003:l89–190.

Girkin, CA. Neuroprotection: Barriers to a breakthrough. *Glaucoma Trials and Tribulations.* American Academy of Ophthalmology. 2003:69–72.

Grajewski, AL. Medical therapy in the pregnant patient. *Glaucoma Trials and Tribulations.* American Academy of Ophthalmology. 2003:109–111.

Johnson DH. Selective laser trabeculoplasty: Is new truly better? *Glaucoma Trials and Tribulations.* American Academy of Ophthalmology. 2003:63–64.

Lewis, RA. The one-site cataract-trabeculectomy combined procedure. *Glaucoma Trials and Tribulations.* American Academy of Ophthalmology. 2003:187–188.

Minckler, D. Ocular blood flow in the glaucoma patient: Is there a meaningful measurement? *Glaucoma Trials and Tribulations.* American Academy of Ophthalmology. 2003:65–67.

Sample, PA. When you should and shouldn't use SWAP. *Glaucoma Trials and Tribulations.* American Academy of Ophthalmology. 2003:5–6.

Shields, MB, Cyclophotocoagulation: Where it fits into glaucoma practice. *Glaucoma Trials and Tribulations.* American Academy of Ophthalmology. 2003:59–62.

Skuta, GL. When one agent fails, should you switch to another in the same class? *Glaucoma Trials and Tribulations.* American Academy of Ophthalmology. 2003:105–106.

Tanaka GH. Is scanning laser imaging of the optic disc a substitute for stereo disc photography? *Glaucoma Trials and Tribulations.* American Academy of Ophthalmology. 2003:51–53.

## GLAUCOMA UNDER PRESSURE: VISION TOWARDS THE FUTURE
American Academy of Ophthalmology Subspecialty Day
(in conjunction with the American Glaucoma Society)
October 19, 2002

Alvarado, JA. Is a computerized optic nerve imaging system essential in glaucoma practice? Yes. *Glaucoma 2002 Under Pressure: Vision Towards the Future.* American Academy of Ophthalmology. 2002:31–36.

Alward, WLM. Molecular genetics on open-angle glaucoma. *Glaucoma 2002 Under Pressure: Vision Towards the Future.* American Academy of Ophthalmology. 2002:121–124.

Asrani, SG. Retinal thickness analyzer. *Glaucoma 2002 Under Pressure: Vision Towards the Future.* American Academy of Ophthalmology. 2002:25–30.

Burgoyne, CF. Is a computerized optic nerve imaging system essential in glaucoma practice? No. *Glaucoma 2002 Under Pressure: Vision Towards the Future.* American Academy of Ophthalmology. 2002:37–39

Chambers, WA. FDA regulations for approval of generics. *Glaucoma 2002 Under Pressure: Vision Towards the Future.* American Academy of Ophthalmology. 2002:63–67.

Coleman, AL. Risk factors for blindness from glaucoma. *Glaucoma 2002 Under Pressure: Vision Towards the Future.* American Academy of Ophthalmology. 2002:41–45.

Garway-Heath, DF. Confocal scanning laser tomography: Taking the measure of glaucomatous optic neuropathy. *Glaucoma 2002 Under Pressure: Vision Towards the Future.* American Academy of Ophthalmology. 2002:9–15.

Greenfield, DS. Scanning laser polarimetry of the RNFL. *Glaucoma 2002 Under Pressure: Vision Towards the Future.* American Academy of Ophthalmology. 2002:17–19.

Herndon, LW. Impact of corneal thickness on glaucoma management. *Glaucoma 2002 Under Pressure: Vision Towards the Future.* American Academy of Ophthalmology. 2002:47–52.

Jost, JB. Clinical assessment of the optic disc and RNFL. *Glaucoma 2002 Under Pressure: Vision Towards the Future.* American Academy of Ophthalmology. 2002:1–7.

McKinnon, SJ. Paradigms for neuroprotection. *Glaucoma 2002 Under Pressure: Vision Towards the Future.* American Academy of Ophthalmology. 2002:109–113.

Schuman, JS. Optical coherence tomography of the RNFL and macula. *Glaucoma 2002 Under Pressure: Vision Towards the Future.* American Academy of Ophthalmology. 2002:21–24.

Wiggs, JL. Molecular genetics of secondary glaucomas. *Glaucoma 2002 Under Pressure: Vision Towards the Future.* American Academy of Ophthalmology. 2002:115–119.

*GLAUCOMA 2001: EVOLUTION AND REVOLUTION*
American Academy of Ophthalmology Subspecialty Day
(in conjunction with the American Glaucoma Society)
November 10, 2001

Anderson, DR. SITA pearls and pitfalls. *Glaucoma 2001: Evolution and Revolution*. American Academy of Ophthalmology. 2001:15–16.

Cantor, LB. Are generic equivalents equivalent? Yes. *Glaucoma 2001: Evolution and Revolution*. American Academy of Ophthalmology. 2001:35–38.

Caprioli, J. What damages the nerve in glaucoma? *Glaucoma 2001: Evolution and Revolution*. American Academy of Ophthalmology. 2001:75–78.

Cioffi, GA. Should NTG be treated differently than POAG? No. *Glaucoma 2001: Evolution and Revolution*. American Academy of Ophthalmology. 2001:143–l 44.

Girkin, CA. Clinical use of SWAP and FDT. *Glaucoma 2001: Evolution and Revolution*. American Academy of Ophthalmology. 2001:17–20.

Greenfield, DS. Are we there yet? Automated detection of progressive structureal injury. *Glaucoma 2001: Evolution and Revolution*. American Academy of Ophthalmology. 2001:9–14.

Gross, RL. Are generic equivalents equivalent? No. *Glaucoma 2001: Evolution and Revolution*. American Academy of Ophthalmology. 2001:39–40.

Higginbotham, EJ. 2001: The new drugs. *Glaucoma 2001: Evolution and Revolution*. American Academy of Ophthalmology. 2001:29–34.

Jampel, HD. Should NTG be treated differently than POAG? Yes. *Glaucoma 2001: Evolution and Revolution*. American Academy of Ophthalmology. 2001:139–141.

Johnstone, MA, Smit, B. What does viscocanalostomy do? *Glaucoma 2001: Evolution and Revolution*. American Academy of Ophthalmology. 2001:187–194.

Mannelli, A. Dissecting Schlemm's Canal in deep sclerectomy.

*Glaucoma 2001: Evolution and Revolution.* American Academy of Ophthalmology. 2001:161–162.

Mermoud, A. Which is the best initial glaucoma procedure? Nonpenetrating surgery. *Glaucoma 2001: Evolution and Revolution.* American Academy of Ophthalmology. 2001:59–60.

Mills, RP. How well does currently available software detect visual field progression? Relatively well. *Glaucoma 2001: Evolution and Revolution.* American Academy of Ophthalmology. 2001:21–22.

Quigley, HA. Do any available drugs provide clinically effective bloodflow or neuroprotection therapy in human glaucoma? *Glaucoma 2001: Evolution and Revolution.* American Academy of Ophthalmology. 2001:89–93.

Realini, AD. Surgical management of neovascular glaucoma. *Glaucoma 2001: Evolution and Revolution.* American Academy of Ophthalmology. 2001:137–138.

Ritch, R. Herbs, potions, and incantations: Alternative therapy and glaucoma. *Glaucoma 2001: Evolution and Revolution.* American Academy of Ophthalmology. 2001:97–102.

Schuman, JS. How well does currently available software detect visual field progression? Not well at all! *Glaucoma 2001: Evolution and Revolution.* American Academy of Ophthalmology. 2001:23–25.

Singh, K. Maximal therapy for glaucoma: When is enough enough? *Glaucoma 2001: Evolution and Revolution.* American Academy of Ophthalmology. 2001:27–28.

Tsai, JC. Surgical approach to malignant glaucoma. *Glaucoma 2001: Evolution and Revolution.* American Academy of Ophthalmology. 2001:125–128.

Wax, MB. Immunologic aspects of glaucoma diagnosis and treatment. *Glaucoma 2001. Evolution and Revolution.* American Academy of Ophthalmology. 2001:73–74.

Werner, EB. Clinical evaluation of NTG. *Glaucoma 2001: Evolution and Revolution.* American Academy of Ophthalmology. 2001:111–115,

Wilson, MR. Should treatment of glaucoma in Blacks differ? *Glaucoma 2001: Evolution and Revolution.* American Academy of Ophthalmology. 2001:47–48.

Wilson RP. Surgical consideration in glaucoma and keratoplasty. *Glaucoma 2001: Evolution and Revolution.* American Academy of Ophthalmology. 2001:129–135.

## AMERICAN GLAUCOMA SOCIETY, FOURTEENTH ANNUAL MEETING
### Final Abstract Book
### Sarasota, Florida. March 2004

Baerveldt G, Ramirez M, Mirhashemi S, Mittelstein M. Surgical outcomes of the trabectome in adult open angle glaucoma—novel surgical device. Abstract #19.

Brown RH, Fellman RL, Ball, SF, Lynch, MG. Eyepass bidirectional glaucoma implant: clinical studies. Abstract #22.

Camras CB, Tois CB, Sjoquist B, et al. Detection of the free acid of bimatoprost in aqueous humor samples from human eyes treated with bimatoprost prior to cataract surgery. Abstract #8.

Kooner, KS. Ex-PRESS glaucoma shunt: Early US experience. Abstract #23.

## AMERICAN GLAUCOMA SOCIETY, THIRTEENTH ANNUAL MEETING
### Final Abstract Book
### San Francisco, California, March 2003

Ahmed IIK. Mitomycin-C augmented deep sclerectomy with collagen wick implantation for high risk glaucoma. Abstract #24.

Alward W. Evaluation of two families with autosomal dominant normal tension glaucoma for mutations in the optimeuron gene. Abstract #1.

Baerveldt GS. Novel glaucoma surgical treatment—goniectomy with histology. Abstract #24.

Friedman DS. Glaucoma prevalence in the United States: Results of a meta-analysis. Abstract #6.

Juzych MS. Comparison of long-term outcome between SLT and ALT in chronic open angle glaucoma patients. Abstract #21.

Kooner KS. Effect of race and gender on central corneal thickness in glaucoma and glaucoma suspect patients. Abstract #10.

Lichter PR. Pigmentary glaucoma: One gene or two? Abstract #2.

Wollstein G. Optical coherence tomography findings predicting future visual field progression. Abstract #12.

# BOOKS

Blumenthal, Mark, Sr. Editor. *The Complete German Commission E Monographs: Therapeutic guide to herbal medicines.* Boston: Integrative Medicine Communications, 1998.

Boyd, Benjamin F, MD, Luntz, Maurice, MD, and Boyd, Samuel MD. *Glaucoma's Etiology. Diagnosis and Management.* Panama, Republic of Panama: Highlights of Ophthalmology, 2002.

Duyff, Roberta Larson. *The American Dietetic Association's Complete Food & Nutrition Guide.* Minneapolis: Chronimed Publishing, 1998.

Eid, Tarek M. and Spaeth, George L. *The Glaucoma's Concepts and Fundamentals.* Philadelphia, PA: Lippincott Williams & Wilkins, 2000.

Epstein, David L. *Chandler and Grant's Glaucoma, Fourth Edition.* Baltimore: Lippincott Williams & Wilkins, 1997.

Goldberg, Stephen. *Ophthalmology Made Ridiculously Simple.* Miami: MedMaster, Inc. 2001.

Grant and Chandler. *Glaucoma.* Philadelphia: Lea & Febiger, 1979.

Gross, Ronald L. *Clinical Glaucoma Management.* Philadelphia: WB Saunders Company, 2001.

Hensyl, William R., Ed. *Stedman's Medical Dictionary.* 25th Ed. Baltimore: Williams & Wilkins, 1990.

Marks, Edith, with Montauredes, Rita. *Coping with Glaucoma.* Garden City Park: Avery Publishing Group, 1997.

*The Medical Advisor: The Complete Guide to Alternative and Conventional Treatments by the Editors of Time-Life Books.* Alexandria: Time-Life Books, 1996.

Morrison, John C, MD, and Pollack, Irvin P., MD. *Glaucoma Science and Practice.* New York: Theme Medical Publishers, Inc., 2003.

*Physicians' Desk Reference (PDR) for Ophthalmic Medicines 2004.* Montvale: Thomson PDR, 2003.

Ritch, Robert, Shields, M. Bruce, Krupin, Theodore. *The Glaucomas, Volumes I and II.* St. Louis: CU Mosby Co., 1989.

Rosenfeld, Isadore. *Dr. Rosenfeld's Guide to Alternative Medicine.* New York: Fawcett Columbine, 1996.

Schattenstein EM. Intraocular pressure and tonometry. In: Ritch R, Shields MB, Krupin T, eds. *The glaucomas. Vol 2. 2nd ed.* St. Louis: CV Mosby, 1996:407–28.

Schulz, Volker, Hänsel, Rudolf, and Tyler, Varro E. *Rational Phytotherapy: A physicians' guide to herbal medicine.* Third Edition. Germany: Springer, 1998.

Shields, M. Bruce. *Textbook of Glaucoma, Fourth Edition.* Philadelphia PA: Lippincott Williams & Wilkins, 2000.

Thomas, John MD. Chief editor. *Glaucoma Surgery.* St. Louis: Mosby-Year Book, Inc., 1992.

Williams AS. Setons in glaucoma surgery. In: Albert DM, Jakobiec FA, Editors. *Principles and practice of ophthalmology: Clinical practice.* Philadelphia: WB Saunders, 1994:1665–1667.

Wilson, MR, Martane, JF. Epidemiology of chronic open-angle glaucoma. In: Ritch R, Shields MB, Krupin T, eds. *The glaucomas. Vol 2. 2nd ed.* St. Louis: CV Mosby, 1996:351–67.

## ONLINE DICTIONARIES

Dorland's Illustrated Medical Dictionary
http://www.mercksource.com/pp/us/cns/cns_hl_dorlands.jspzQz pgzEzzSzppdocszSzuszSz . . .
Medline Plus Medical Dictionary
www.nlm.nih.gov/medlineplus/mplusdictionary.html
Medterms.com Medical Dictionary
www.medterms.com
Merriam Webster Medical Dictionary ©2003 by Merriam-Webster, Inc.
www.intellihealth.com

# WEB SITES

The Glaucoma Foundation
www.glaucomafoundation.org
American Academy of Ophthalmology
www.aao.org
American Glaucoma Society
www.glaucomanet.org
Glaucoma Research Foundation
www.glaucoma.org
Lighthouse International
www.lighthouse.org
Alcon Laboratories Inc. USA
www.alcon/US/
Allergan USA
www.allergan.com
Carl Zeiss Meditec, Inc.
www.humphrey.com
Cosopt
www.cosopt.com
Lumenis
www.lumenis.com
Lumigan
www.lumigan.com
Travatan
www.travatan.com
Xalatan
www.xalatan.com
VisionCare Ophthalmic Technologies
www.visioncareinc.net
Online Mendelian Inheritance in Man (OMIM)
www.ncbi.nlm.nih.gov/entrez/query.fcgi?db-OMIM/
American Dietetic Association. Antioxidant Vitamins for Optimal Health.
www.eatright.org.

# NEWSLETTERS

"Doheny/USC Researchers Spearhead $17 Million Biomimetics Project" Update: Doheny Eye Institute. Vol 19 No. 2. Winter 2004.

"First genetic marker for glaucoma found." Eye to Eye: The Newsletter of The Glaucoma Foundation, Vol 12, No. 1, Spring 2001.

"Novel mechanism of cell death uncovered." Eye to Eye: The Newsletter of The Glaucoma Foundation, Vol 12, No. 1, Spring 2001.

"On the road to gene-based therapy" Eye to Eye: The Newsletter of The Glaucoma Foundation, Vol 12, No. 1, Spring 2001.

"Glaucoma and aerobic exercise" Eye to Eye: The Newsletter of The Glaucoma Foundation, Vol 12, No. 1, Spring 2001.

Glaucoma Foundation Newsletter, Winter 2003, Glaucoma and Pregnancy—What you should know!

"Alternative medicine and you: Part 1 of a 2-part series." Gleams Newsletter, Glaucoma Research Foundation, Summer 1999, Vol 17, No 1.

"Nutrition and Glaucoma: Part 2 of a 2-part series." Gleams Newsletter, Glaucoma Research Foundation, Fall 1999, Vol 17, No. 2.

# Index

# ABOUT THE AUTHORS

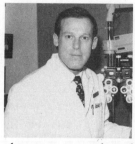 **Gregory K. Harmon, M.D.**, is associate professor of clinical ophthalmology at Weill Medical College of Cornell University and director of the Glaucoma Service at New York Presbyterian Hospital. Dr. Harmon is chairman and CEO of The Glaucoma Foundation, the nation's foremost nonprofit organization promoting glaucoma research and awareness.

Dr. Harmon is a graduate of The Johns Hopkins University and Mount Sinai School of Medicine. He completed his internship in internal medicine at St. Luke's-Roosevelt Hospital, and his residency in ophthalmology and fellowship in glaucoma at Cornell Medical Center.

An experienced spokesperson and advocate for widespread glaucoma screening, Dr. Harmon has produced and been featured in news segments and public service announcements that have achieved national distribution on television and radio. He has also conducted glaucoma screenings among high-profile populations, such as the NY Yankees and Mets, and in large corporations such as NBC. Dr. Harmon has written patient-education guides and contributed to numerous textbooks and medical journals.


**Nancy Intrator** is a freelance writer specializing in health and family-related topics, and is co-author (with Hugh Melnick, M.D.) of *The Pregnancy Prescription*, a consumer book on infertility.

Ms. Intrator was editor and chief contributor for *Food & Fitness Advisor*, the nationally distributed fitness and nutrition newsletter affiliated with The Center for Women's Healthcare, Weill Medical College of Cornell University. Her articles have appeared in *Cos-*

mopolitan, *American Health*, *Avenue*, *Working Mother*, *The Christian Science Monitor*, *Yachting*, *Offshore Magazine*, *Westchester/New York/Long Island Family*, and specialized publications in the health-care industry. Ms. Intrator has a B.A. from the University of Pennsylvania and an M.B.A. from Columbia Business School.

Nancy Intrator's husband was diagnosed with glaucoma in his thirties. Because of her personal experience, she is committed to increasing awareness and understanding of all aspects of this disease among the general public.

**OTHER TITLES FROM THE BESTSELLING SERIES
WHAT YOUR DOCTOR MAY *NOT* TELL YOU ABOUT™ ...**

## AUTOIMMUNE DISORDERS
The Revolutionary Drug-free Treatments for Thyroid
Disease · Lupus · MS · IBD · Chronic Fatigue ·
Rheumatoid Arthritis, and Other Diseases

## BREAST CANCER
How Hormone Balance Can Help Save Your Life

## CHILDREN'S ALLERGIES AND ASTHMA
Simple Steps to Help Stop Attacks and
Improve Your Child's Health

## CHILDREN'S VACCINATIONS
Learn What You Should—and Should Not—Do to Protect
Your Kids

## CIRCUMCISION
Untold Facts on America's Most Widely Performed—
and Most Unnecessary—Surgery

## FIBROIDS
New Techniques and Therapies—Including
Breakthrough Alternatives

## FIBROMYALGIA
The Revolutionary Treatment That Can Reverse
the Disease

*more ...*

### FIBROMYALGIA FATIGUE
The Powerful Program That Helps
You Boost Your Energy and Reclaim Your Life

### HIP AND KNEE REPLACEMENT SURGERY
Everything You Need to Know
to Make the Right Decisions

### HPV AND ABNORMAL PAP SMEARS
Get the Facts on This Dangerous Virus—Protect Your
Health and Your Life!

### HYPERTENSION
The Revolutionary Nutrition and Lifestyle Program to
Help Fight High Blood Pressure

### HYPOTHYROIDISM
A Simple Plan for Extraordinary Results

### IBS
Eliminate Your Symptoms and Live a Pain-free,
Drug-free Life

### KNEE PAIN AND SURGERY
Learn the Truth About MRIs and Common Misdiagnoses—
and Avoid Unnecessary Surgery

### MENOPAUSE
The Breakthrough Book on *Natural* Hormone Balance

### MIGRAINES
The Breakthrough Program That Can Help End Your Pain

*copy p. 28*

## OSTEOPOROSIS
Help Prevent—and Even Reverse—the Disease
That Burdens Millions of Women

## PARKINSON'S DISEASE
A Holistic Program for Optimal Wellness

## PEDIATRIC FIBROMYALGIA
A Safe, New Treatment Plan for Children

## PREMENOPAUSE
Balance Your Hormones and Your Life
from Thirty to Fifty

## SINUSITIS
Relieve Your Symptoms and Identify
the Real Source of Your Pain

Humphrey Automated perimeter
visual field testing pp 122-125